T0144740

BASIC HEALTH PUBLICATIONS USER'S GUIDE

TO

NATURAL HORMONE REPLACEMENT

Learn How Safe Dietary
& Herbal Supplements
Can Ease Your
Midlife Changes.

KATHLEEN BARNES

JACK CHALLEM Series Editor

The information contained in this book is based upon the research and personal and professional experiences of the author. It is not intended as a substitute for con-sulting with your physician or other healthcare provider. Any attempt to diagnose and treat an illness should be done under the direction of a healthcare professional. The publisher does not advocate the use of any particular healthcare protocol but believes the information in this book should be available to the public. The publisher and author are not responsible for any adverse effects or consequences resulting from the use of the suggestions, preparations, or procedures discussed in this book. Should the reader have any questions con-cerning the appropriateness of any procedures or preparations mentioned, the author and the publisher strongly suggest consulting a professional healthcare advisor.

Series Editor: Jack Challem
Editor: Jane Morrill
Typesetter: Theresa Wiscovitch
Series Cover Designer: Mike Stromberg

Basic Health Publications User's Guides are published by Basic Health Publications, Inc.

ISBN: 978-1-59120-171-7 (Pbk.)
ISBN: 978-1-68162-863-9 (Hardcover)

CONTENTS

Introduction, 1

1. Perimenopause: New Beginnings, 4

2. Your Changing Body, 9

3. Finding the Right Doctor, 13

4. Conventional Medicine's Approach, 21

5. Dealing with Menopausal Symptoms, 24

6. Postmenopause: A Woman's Needs, 27

7. A Suitable Diet, 36

8. The Best Exercise, 44

9. Natural Herbs and Supplements, 50

10. Stress Management, Meditation, and More, 67

11. Bioidentical Hormone Replacement, 76

Conclusion, 83

Selected References, 84

Other Books and Resources, 87

Index, 89

INTRODUCTION

Our mothers and grandmothers whispered the words, "The Change." We could hear the capital letters. We could hear the dread in their voices. If we watched carefully, we could see the older women exchange knowing nods of sympathy and then quickly change the subject.

Until the past decade or so, menopause and perimenopause were subjects of deep dark mystery. Medical science knew little about "The Change" that will eventually affect all women. The women of our mothers' or grandmothers' era had only the word-of-mouth exchanged over countless cups of tea and chats over the back fence. Only with a generation of Baby Boomers who demand answers and results has menopause become a topic of popular discussion and increasing medical research.

In the mid-1900s, when scientists and the pharmaceutical industry discovered that the urine of all mammals contained estrogen, a new industry was born. Placid pregnant mares were an easy source, and from their urine, hormone replacement drugs were made that remain conventional medicine's treatment of choice for the symptoms of menopause.

Millions of women found relief from the hot flashes, mood swings, insomnia, night sweats, and short-term memory loss that often go hand-in-hand with the approach of menopause. Doctors told women they'd need to take these drugs for a lifetime—and assured them that the estrogen in synthetic hormone replacement would protect them against heart attacks, strokes, cancer, and Alzheimer's disease.

We now know that this information is 180 degrees from the truth. In 2002, more than fifty years after equine-based hormone replacement therapy (HRT) went on the market, the Women's Health Initiative, a large clinical study, brought the truth out once and for all. Equine-based HRT combined with synthetic progesterone offered no protection at all from those dread diseases. In fact, it actually *increased* the risk of heart attack by 27 percent and the risk of stroke by 38 percent. Women taking these drugs more than doubled their risk of blood clots.

If that wasn't bad enough, later results of the study released in 2004 showed that the drugs also increased the risk of dementia and other neurological illnesses such as Alzheimer's disease by a stunning 105 percent. And the drugs increased the risk of type 2 diabetes by 21 percent.

The medical profession was in a dither. Many women stopped taking their equine-based hormone replacement drugs cold-turkey, throwing their bodies into hormone swings that, by comparison, made the early phases of menopausal hot flashes seem like a Sunday School picnic. Sadly, the vast majority of doctors are still basically clueless about natural ways to address menopause. Even more sadly, their patients haven't had the benefit of gentle and natural ways to approach this natural life transition.

Today, 40 million American women are somewhere in the process of menopause. By 2015, 60 million of us will be in menopause and perimeno - pause and half of all American women will be at some point in "The Change." The sheer weight of those numbers has forced medical science and society in general to re-examine a subject that was once a scientific backwater.

This new knowledge and the new openness about this women's mystery are welcome. However, we are discovering that our foremothers had many of the answers to the issues of menopause in their herb cabinets. This book is intended to help you understand what's happening in your body as hormone levels begin to fluctuate, and to give you a menu of natural ways to relieve your symptoms and improve your long-term health and longevity. If you've been taking equine-based HRT, you'll learn how to safely withdraw from the drugs and replace them with harmless, healthy natural alternatives.

So, curl up with a steaming cup of herbal tea, and read away. Your body will thank you!

CHAPTER 1

PERIMENOPAUSE: NEW BEGINNINGS

Perimenopause is the phase between the beginning of hormonal changes and full menopause, which is medically defined as the absence of menstrual periods for twelve months. Technically, perimenopause begins when your ovulation becomes irregular because your ovaries have released just about all the viable eggs with which you were born. It signals an alteration in your body's natural production of two essential hormones: estrogen and progesterone.

Throughout your life, your pituitary gland sends signals to your ovaries to produce more estrogen. Sometimes, your ovaries respond to the message, and sometimes, as you get older, they don't. As a result, in perimenopause your estrogen levels fluctuate by the month, by the day, and even by the hour. Fluctuating estrogen and falling progesterone levels can cause a variety of annoying symptoms ranging from the dreaded hot flashes, to butt-of-male-jokes irritability and mood swings, to debilitating hormonal headaches, depression, and joint pain.

Perimenopause
The period before menopause, characterized by hormonal fluctuations.

The list of symptoms is long. Each woman's perimenopause is unique. Some women sail through it with barely noticeable symptoms, while others suffer in the extreme. Most women fall somewhere in the middle, with one or two symptoms becoming particularly bothersome. The most common perimenopausal symptoms are:

- Depression
- Erratic menstrual cycles
- Hot flashes
- Night sweats
- Insomnia
- Palpitations
- Mood swings
- Extraordinarily heavy or light periods
- Short-term memory loss
- Increased growth of facial hair

- Irritability
- Joint pain
- Hormonal headaches
- Food cravings and weight gain
- Vaginal dryness and itching
- Loss of hair on the head
- Loss of skin elasticity
- Loss of interest in sex

While these symptoms are annoying and occasionally cause a serious change in a woman's quality of life, they are generally not life-threatening. However, the long-term effects of declining hormones can contribute to much more serious health problems, ranging from heart disease to osteoporosis, dental and periodontal changes, urinary incontinence, and hormone-related malignancies, such as breast, ovarian, and endometrial cancers.

The Change before "The Change"

Perimenopausal symptoms can begin by the time a woman reaches her mid-thirties, although most commonly they begin in the mid to late forties. Just as American girls are reaching puberty at increasingly early ages, women are finding that meno-pause can begin early, too. Experts theorize that this may be due to high levels of hormones in our food supply, particularly the hormones fed to livestock and consumed in dairy and meat products. The average age for menopause in the United States is fifty or fifty-one. It may come sooner for women who took birth-control pills for extended periods of time.

How Long Will It Take?

That's the $64,000 question! For some women, perimenopause begins just a few months before full menopause. However, for most women, it starts as hormone levels begin to drop and continues over a long period of time. For some women, the perimenopausal process can take as long as ten years. Fortunately, for most of us, the most intense parts of the process only last a year or two.

It's Not a Disease

Menopause is not a disease, although it's often treated as one by conventional medicine. Menopause is a natural, healthy process by which the female human body ends the reproductive years. Of course, the most obvious change during menopause is a gradual cessation of a woman's ability to become pregnant.

Natural health expert Shari Lieberman, Ph.D., in her book, *Get Off the Menopause Roller Coaster*, calls this time a blessing. "This, friends, is something to be grateful for, rather than to resist. Do you really want to be pregnant in your fifties or sixties?"

Conventional medicine is also quick to prescribe conjugated equine estrogens (made from the urine of pregnant horses) to relieve the symptoms of per-

---

You just might be in perimenopause . . .

- if your periods were always as regular as clockwork and suddenly they're way off course.

- if you're spotting between periods.

- if your periods have suddenly become very heavy, very light, or both.

---

imenopause. In light of the results of the Women's Health Initiative, this type of hormone replacement has been found to be an unwise path for almost every woman.

It's Not All in Your Head

A mercifully dwindling element of the medical profession wants us to think that symptoms of perimenopause and menopause are largely psychological—hence, the word "hysterectomy," implying a condition promoted by hysteria. However, the roller-coaster ride of perimenopausal symptoms is no Sunday School picnic. The hormone fluctuations alone can lead to what may appear to be psychological symptoms—irritability, mood swings, and depression. It's not surprising that many women feel overwhelmed by the changes taking place in their bodies at this time. But if your doctor tries to tell you that your symptoms are all in your head, look for another doctor, one who understands what's happening in your body and knows how to treat it.

The Spiritual Element

There is a spiritual element of menopause not often recognized in our Western culture. This is the concept of "elderhood," or the archetypal wise woman. As Clarissa Pinkola Estes says in *Women Who Run with the Wolves*, the elder women should be honored simply because they have lived so long.

In ancient times, only extremely long-lived women survived long enough to reach menopause. Crones were revered by their families and tribes for their wisdom, their powers of discrimination, and their sage leadership. Today, the age of menopause is little more than a midpoint in a woman's life. It doesn't signal old age; rather, it is a sign that a woman is making a transition from the motherhood years to a new stage of life characterized by freedom from the responsibilities of child rearing and the fear of pregnancy, a loosening of sexual inhibitions, and the blossoming of creative energies.

Ann Kreilkamp, founder of *Crone Chronicles*, sums up the spiritual aspects of the modern woman's transition through menopause. She says, "For the first time in history, enormous numbers of women are traveling through the gate of menopause and looking forward to a life span of some thirty more years. And we women have a certain hard-won wisdom gleaned through consciously processing the experiences of our long and fruitful lives. What are we going to do with this wisdom? Play golf? Get our hair done? We begin to glimpse the opportunity and the responsibility."

Kreilkamp continues, "To evaluate the Crone stage of life consciously is to see this phase as the crowning glory, the time when a woman enters into her full maturity, inside and out. By this new (and very ancient) measure, the Crone is the most revered stage of life, rather than the least; she is the most honored, not the most ignored. Distilling wisdom from experience, her words, attitudes, and actions can now serve as examples to others."

CHAPTER 2

YOUR CHANGING BODY

Our greatest fear is the unknown. Perhaps that's why our mothers and grandmothers dreaded "The Change" so much. The body of research that has emerged in the past decade or two reflects, among other things, modern woman's demands to understand what's happening in her body and to find ways to address the symptoms of perimenopause and menopause.

It's Not Just Nose-Diving Estrogen

Perimenopause is not a simple matter of nose-diving estrogen production. One of the first clinical signs of menopause is a gradual decline in progesterone levels.

At the same time, estrogen levels may remain stable or even increase slightly. To further complicate matters, estrogen is actually a group of several hormones, any one of which can become unbalanced.

Progesterone and estrogen play a delicate balancing act throughout the menstrual cycle, rising and falling as the cycle progresses. Without sufficient progesterone, estrogen becomes dominant. Here's an explanation of what Marla Ahlgrimm calls "the estrogen/ progesterone *pas de deux*" in her book, *The HRT Solution*:

Progesterone

A natural hormone made by the ovaries that sustains pregnancy, nurtures the fertilized egg, and helps your body manufacture estrogen and testosterone.

- Estrogen causes an increase in endometrial cell

production; progesterone protects the endometrium from this kind of cell growth.

- Estrogen suppresses the action of the thyroid gland; progesterone enhances it.

- Estrogen increases salt and fluid retention; progesterone works like a diuretic, prompting the body to excrete fluids.

Estrogen
The major female hormone, which is composed of three predominant hormones: estriol, estradiol, and estrone.

The uncomfortable symptoms of perimenopause are actually the result of an excess of estrogen. So, for most women, estrogen-based hormone replacement alone isn't helpful at all. As a woman moves further into perimenopause, progesterone continues its decline, while estrogen levels begin to swing like a pendulum and instead of releasing one mature egg, the ovaries begin to release whole groups of mature eggs each month. The early signs of declining progesterone levels are:

- Breast swelling

- Heavy menstrual bleeding

- Irregular periods

- Premenstrual headaches

- Water retention

- Weight gain around the abdomen and hips

At the same time, we begin to see the seesawing levels of follicle-stimulating hormone (FSH) and luteinizing hormone (LH), the hormones that are normally released by the pituitary gland to help the egg mature and regulate ovulation. As you approach full menopause, your FSH and LH levels will stabilize and remain stable for the rest of your life.

That's an important point: These crazy hormonal swings are temporary. There's no telling exactly how long the process of perimenopause will last, but when it's over, it's over!

Three Types of Menopause

Perimenopause has been compared to climbing up a mountain. There are three ways to get to the top, says Dr. Christiane Northrup, author of *The Wisdom of Menopause*:

1. Natural menopause (climbing the sloping, winding path to the top), which occurs gradually, usually between the ages of forty-five and fifty-five.

2. Premature menopause (the short path straight to the top of the mountain) that takes place early for a variety of reasons, including an illness such as an autoimmune disease, a nutritional deficiency, or chronic stress (including excessive athletic conditioning).

3. Artificial menopause (a helicopter ride to the top that doesn't give your body a chance to acclimatize itself to the changing landscape), which takes place abruptly because of the surgical removal of any part of the reproductive system, radiation or chemotherapy, or certain drugs that mimic menopause for medical reasons.

Toxic Estrogen

Not only can too much estrogen be toxic to your body, but there are increasing numbers of toxic estrogens present in our environment and they can increase the incidence of unbalanced hormones or estrogen dominance. These hormones, called "xeno - estrogens," mimic the effect of estrogen when they are taken into the human body, causing, among other things, rapid cell growth in breast tissue.

Xenoestrogens have been implicated in a wide variety of human maladies ranging from infertility and endometriosis to breast and ovarian cancers. They accumulate in the fatty tissues of the body and the breast of a convenient target. Unfortun - ately, the fatty tissues of the animals we eat are also repositories for xenoestrogens. Some experts believe that they increase the severity of perimenopausal symptoms in modern women. Xenoestrogens can be found in:

- Drugs, such as diethylstilbestrol (DES), a medication given to millions of pregnant American women between 1948 and 1972 to prevent miscarriages.

- Emissions from coal-burning power plants and automobile-exhaust pipes.

- Heavy metals, including mercury, lead, and cadmium, used in the manufacture of batteries, paints, fluorescent lighting fixtures, paints, fossil fuels, dental amalgams, and other ubiquitous products in our daily lives.

- Pesticides, herbicides, and insecticides, including dichloro-diphenyl-trichloromethane (DDT), a pesticide banned in 1983 that still exists in residual levels in our soil and is still in use outside the United States. Endosulphan, an insecticide that has not been banned, and altrazine, the most commonly used weed killer in American cornfields, are also xenoestrogens.

- Plastics and the chemicals used in their manufacture, including nonylphenol, a chemical added during the manufacture of plastic to prevent it from cracking. Nonylphenol is also an additive in many pesticides, detergents, and spermicides. Bisphenol A, a byproduct of plastic manufacturing and the breakdown of food-can linings and juice packaging, is another potent xenoestrogen.

If you've had extensive exposure to xenoestrogens, they may affect your body in general and the process of your perimenopause and menopause in particular. Armed with this information about your present hormonal status and the possibility of external factors that may be influencing perimeno - pause, you should now be ready to discuss your options with your healthcare provider.

CHAPTER 3

FINDING THE RIGHT DOCTOR

You may have noticed the attitudes of conventional medicine toward so-called "alternative" or "complementary" approaches to perimeno-pause, menopause, and the testing for conditions associated with both. I do not intend to become involved in doctor-bashing or scorn for conventional medicine. Conventional medicine is enormously helpful and often necessary.

Many conventional doctors, however, are not as up to date as they could be, particularly when it comes to the growing body of research on peri-menopause and menopause. Many others are simply unaware that there are natural approaches to menopause that have been used by women for thousands of years. There are even natural forms of hormone replacement that have been available in the United States for forty years or more.

Few conventional doctors receive training in medical school or beyond on the powers of proper nutrition to address dozens of medical conditions. Some are biased against natural approaches and may actually ridicule you when you ask about them. And, sadly, some are susceptible to the arguments of drug-company representatives.

Educate Your Doctor

That leaves it up to you to educate your doctor. Fortunately, you're not alone like your mother and grandmother were. There is abundant material available in the medical literature, in books, and on websites. Doctors of great renown, such as Dr.

Christiane Northrup, Dr. John Lee, Dr. Jonathan Wright, clinical nutritionist Dr. Shari Lieberman, naturopathic physician Dr. Marcus Laux, pharmacist Dr. Marla Ahlgrimm, and many others have written authoritative books to help educate you and your doctor on natural approaches to perimenopause. See the Other Books and Resources section for full details of their work.

Many experts consider Dr. Wright's slim volume, *Natural Hormone Replacement for Women Over 45*, to be one of the simplest and most persuasive books for both patients and doctors. Make an appointment with your doctor to discuss your symptoms and concerns.

You may be lucky and have a doctor who's on top of the game—or not. If you've done your homework in advance, you may be able to offer some simple research or a book to help bring your doctor up to speed. You might offer your doctor a copy of this book or some of the books listed in the Other Books and Resources section. If your doctor is resistant to anything but the conventional Premarin/Provera/Fosamax approach to perimenopause, consider finding another doctor. The Other Books and Resources section can help you find the right doctor, too.

Premarin, Provera, and Fosamax
Synthetic drugs designed to replace estrogen and progesterone and prevent bone loss.

Figuring Out Where You Are

Your hormone profile is as unique as your fingerprint. It can change by the month, by the day, and even by the hour. The only way you and your doctor can determine your true hormone status is by testing levels of the major hormones and retesting them every few months.

Estrogen

Estrogen is actually a blanket term for three distinct

hormones: estrone, estradiol, and estriol. These three types of estrogen are protective against a grab bag of health issues ranging from osteoporosis to heart disease, Alzheimer's disease, colon cancer, urinary incontinence, and even tooth decay. European research suggests estriol may also protect against other forms of cancer. Proper estrogen balance enhances sleep, mood, mental sharpness and memory, digestion, sex drive, skin tone, and brain chemistry, including the feel-good endorphins and serotonin.

Progesterone

This hormone is produced by the ovaries after ovulation, with levels increasing in the second half of the menstrual cycle. Progesterone is necessary for fertility and maintaining pregnancy. At perimenopause, progesterone can have a calming effect. It regulates fluid balances to prevent bloating, increases energy and sex drive, and stabilizes blood sugar, thyroid function, and mineral balance. Progesterone has also been shown to decrease the risk of cancer of the endometrium (uterine lining) and may help to protect against breast cancer, fibrocystic breasts, and osteoporosis.

Testosterone

Testosterone isn't just a male hormone; women have it, too, and it is the hormone of desire in both sexes. Natural testosterone levels diminish during perimenopause, although the ovaries and adrenal glands continue to produce small amounts. This offers at least a partial explanation for the declining sexual desire that many women experience as perimenopause progresses. Testosterone helps with tissue growth and stimulates blood flow. It can also help to relieve perimenopausal symptoms, including depression, bone-density loss, and diminished sex drive.

DHEA

This tongue twister, dehydroepiandrosterone, has been called the "fountain of youth" hormone. Although DHEA is manufactured by the adrenal glands, skin, and brain, not by the ovaries, natural levels of this important hormone decline as we age. It can help our bodies produce adequate amounts of estrogen and testosterone. Having sufficient DHEA enhances immune function and sex drive, elevates mood, improves insulin function, and may even lower cholesterol. It also helps to lower levels of the stress hormone, cortisol.

Cortisol

Known as the stress hormone, cortisol is released during prolonged periods of stress. It also helps to regulate the way the body metabolizes protein and carbohydrates, which is why it is often associated with stress-related weight gain. Elevated cortisol levels can lead to high blood sugar and impair the body's ability to use protein properly, indirectly leading to muscle-wasting and osteoporosis. Too much cortisol has also been shown to impair memory.

However, cortisol also has a positive side. It's important for good immune function, strong blood vessels, and muscle function.

The Best Tests

There are lab tests for the levels of all the above hormones; however, insurance companies may balk at requests for testing that goes beyond estrogen, progesterone, and testosterone.

Your hormone levels can be tested either with a saliva test or a blood test. Physicians on the cutting edge of the natural menopause movement prefer saliva testing because it is the most reliable way to determine free or unbound hormone levels. This has been known for more than thirty years, although most physicians are unaware of it. The saliva test is easier for the patient, because the test kit is sent home and samples can be collected at several times during the day.

Some laboratories will conduct these tests without a doctor's prescription, but they are most commonly performed under a doctor's orders. If you have problems finding a cooperative doctor, please see the Other Books and Resources section.

Blood tests for free or unbound hormone levels are similar to a host of other blood tests frequently ordered by doctors. The major drawback of blood testing is the daily fluctuation of hormones, and the sample is taken only once, usually at a time that is convenient to the doctor's office or the lab.

What Your Results Mean

When you get your test results, you'll have a snapshot of your hormonal profile at a given time in your perimenopausal journey. Here are the normal ranges for the most common tests:

- **Estradiol.** This is the major marker of your most important estrogen component. Normal range for nonmenopausal women on day 14 of their menstrual cycles is 150–170 pg/ml (picograms per milliliter). For menopausal women, normal is less than 20 pg/ml.

- **Progesterone.** Normal range is 0.2–28 ng/ml (nanograms per milliliter) for nonmenopausal women and 0–0.7 ng/ml for menopausal women.

- **Total testosterone.** Normal range is 14–76 ng/dl for nonmenopausal women and 5–51 ng/dl (nanograms per deciliter) for menopausal women.

If you've chosen to do the DHEA and cortisol tests, here are the normal ranges:

- **DHEA.** Normal range for women aged nineteen to thirty is 29–781 mcg/dl (micrograms per deciliter); for women aged thirty-one to fifty it is 12–379 mcg/dl; and for postmenopausal women it's 30–260 mcg/dl.

• **Cortisol.** Normal range for a test taken in the morning is 4.3–22.4 mcg/dl. For an evening test, normal range is 3.1–16.7 mcg/dl.

Finding your hormone levels will help you and your doctor make some decisions about where you are in the menopausal process and how to address the symptoms, as well as the long-term effects that accompany it.

Thyroid and Perimenopause

You might also consider thyroid function testing, since epidemiological evidence shows that 26 percent of women in or near perimenopause have low thyroid function (hypothyroidism). Hypothyroidism and estrogen dominance have been linked by several studies. However, laboratory tests may not be conclusive since an estimated 30 percent of perimenopausal women have sub-clinical hypothyroidism or low thyroid function that doesn't show up on blood tests. Dr. Christiane Northrup says that this is because the thyroid is functioning properly, but the excess free estrogen that accompanies menopause is blocking the thyroid hormones from working effectively.

Even if they may not show the true picture of your thyroid function, blood tests can give you a starting point. You should have the standard TSH (thyroid-stimulating hormone) tests. Normal range is considered to be between 0.35 and 5.5 mu/ml (microunits per milliliter). The optimal level is under 2. If you are above 2, you may have an underactive thyroid gland, but most doctors think you need a higher result to be considered hypothyroid. Most doctors stop with the TSH test, but you can obtain more information from these tests.

- **T4 (total thyroxine).** Normal range is 4.5–12.0 ug/dl (micrograms per deciliter). A reading of less than 4.5 with a high TSH may indicate hypothyroidism.

- **Free T4.** Normal range is between 0.7 and 1.53 ug/dl (micrograms per deciliter). Less than 0.7 may indicate hypothyroidism.

- **Total T3 (triiodothyronine).** This measures the thyroid hormone that circulates in your blood. Normal range is 60–181 ng/dl. Less than 60 ng/dl may indicate hypothyroidism. An optimal reading is 120–124 ng/dl.

- **Free T3.** Normal range is approximately 260–480 pg/ml; less than 260 pg/ml may indicate hypothyroidism.

Low Thyroid Function

Even if your thyroid tests come back within normal ranges, however, you may have hypothyroidism. There are dozens of symptoms, and any one or two of them could indicate a need for thyroid hormone supplementation. Among the symptoms are:

- Fatigue and weakness

- Weight gain

- Difficulty losing weight

- Cold extremities

- Irritability

- Thinning hair

- Eyebrows thinning or disappearing at the outer edges

- Coarse, dry skin

- Depression

- Memory loss

- Irregular menstrual cycles

Notice the remarkable similarity between these symptoms and the signs of perimenopause. That's not an accident; the two conditions are intimately intertwined.

The Insurance Hurdle

You have one last obstacle to overcome: your insurance company. You may have already stumbled a little on this one. Many insurance companies won't cover saliva testing, and you may have to pay for your prescriptions yourself. Saliva testing typically costs about $60.

If you can get your doctor to send a letter of medical necessity to your insurance company, explaining that the care you need is not available within the existing scope of the plan, you may get some help. You may need to write a letter to your insurance company yourself, becoming an advocate and an educator again. If worse comes to worst, you can simply pay the costs of the test yourself, knowing you're getting the best possible information.

CHAPTER 4

CONVENTIONAL MEDICINE'S APPROACH

Now that your tests have confirmed that you are perimenopausal, it's time to make some decisions about the next step. Will you choose conventional medicine, or will you go natural? If you decide to try herbs and supplements, see Chapter 9. If you decide to take the diet and exercise route, check out Chapters 7 and 8. If you decide you need some form of hormone replacement, Chapter 11 will point you in the right direction. If, however, you choose conventional medicine, there are some things you should be aware of.

Warning!

If you're like many women entering "The Change," your doctor may tell you it's time for Premarin, a horse-urine-based system of estrogen delivery, or PremPro, a combination of Premarin and a syn-thetic form of progesterone usually prescribed for women who have had hysterectomies. Fortunately, fewer doctors are recommending equine-based hormone replacement in the aftermath of the Women's Health Initiative, which clearly demonstrated the dangers of taking hormones that are not relevant to the human system.

Just Say, "Neigh"

If your doctor does recommend synthetic hormone replacement consider this: Women aren't horses. Our hormonal makeup is vastly different. Although horse-urine estrogen may be effective in easing some of the more unpleasant symptoms of menopause, the science is now solid: It increases your risk of serious illness. In three words: Don't take it! Dr. Jonathan Wright once said, "The next time I see a menopausal horse, I will be happy to prescribe Premarin, a horse estrogen!"

Synthetic Estrogen

Table 4.1 contains an interesting comparison between the estrogen balance of a typical adult woman and the contents of Premarin (PREgnant MAres' uRINe), the leading brand of what the drug industry calls "conjugated equine estrogens."

TABLE 4.1.		
Types of Estrogen	**Women**	**Premarin**
Estrone	10 to 20 percent	80 percent
Estradiol	10 to 20 percent	Trace amounts
Estriol	60 to 80 percent	0 percent
Equilin	0 percent	20 percent

Estradiol
The most potent form of estrogen and the most commonly implicated in increased cancer risk.

Much of the pharmaceutical hormone replacement therapy (HRT) is 100 percent estradiol, the most potent form of estrogen, of which women naturally have only about 20 percent.

Neither estradiol nor Premarin is an ideal match, and neither even remotely resembles the hormonal makeup of the human female. It's no wonder that these compounds have played havoc with women's health for fifty years!

Synthetic Progesterone

Clearly, there are health dangers in Premarin and PremPro or progestin, a synthetic form of progesterone. For some women, doctors decide to prescribe progestin. Progestin and progesterone are as different as night and day. Progestin has been linked to a large number of side effects, including heart disease, increased depression and mood swings, strokes, uterine cancer, and water retention.

Natural progesterone, on the other hand, actually protects against uterine cancer. It also helps build strong bones and helps create other hormones when they are needed.

Getting Off the Mare-Y-Go-Round

If you've been taking equine-based hormones, or any hormones, for that matter, you can always stop. But do it gradually. If you suddenly stop taking any of these medications, your body will be thrown into a complete hormonal turmoil. Hot flashes from hell, mood swings that can border on clinical depression, and other equally unpleasant symptoms can make your life miserable. Take it slowly.

Talk to your doctor about your desire to get off the mare-y-go-round, but don't be surprised if you meet resistance or an insistence that you will need an anti-osteoporosis drug to prevent the "inevitable" bone loss that comes from the loss of these hormones. Osteoporosis is not inevitable, especially if you're physically active (see Chapter 8).

Don't Go Cold Turkey

But you will need to taper off horse-based hormones over the course of several months. Since the capsules can't be cut in half, the best advice is to cut back to taking them every other day. After a couple of months, assuming that your symptoms haven't become intolerable, take a pill every third day. If that's still okay, after a couple of months take one every fourth day, and so on until you're taking only one a week. Then, if you still have no real problems, you can stop.

This process may take eight or nine months. If hot flashes and insomnia or other symptoms begin, you might want to try taking black cohosh, vitex, or another supplement (see Chapter 9). It's best to work hand in hand with your doctor on this process if your doctor is willing.

CHAPTER 5

DEALING WITH MENOPAUSAL SYMPTOMS

L uckily for most of us, the annoyances of peri-menopause, however numerous and uncom-fortable, are short term. In the long term, however, there are considerations of heart health and other important health concerns that you'll need to address. All of this may seem daunting, especially if you're feeling a bit fragile in the face of these changes in your body, mind, and spirit. The coming chapters will provide ways to address this batch of annoying symptoms easily, safely, and naturally.

There are dozens of options open to you that can help you to live an active life well into your eighties, nineties, or beyond. The choices are yours. Many women do well with special attention to diet and exercise. Others opt for natural hormone replacement for a few years. Some opt to keep the hormones flowing over the long term.

Defining your goals will help you make those choices. If you think you can turn back the aging process and stay young forever, you will be disappointed with any approach you choose to deal with your menopause. Denying the natural aging process is fruitless. However, addressing your peri-menopause sensibly, and then gracefully entering late middle age and old age is not only possible, it's what most of us choose to do.

Does this mean you have to put on an ankle-length black dress and sit rocking on the porch for the next thirty years? Not a chance! Have you noticed that women in general are staying active and healthy later in life?

Healthy Old Age

Think of your grandmother or your great-grandmother, if you were lucky enough to know her. It's likely that they were old ladies when they were in their sixties and seventies. If they were "proper ladies" of their time, exercise was practically unheard of, and fresh fruits and vegetables were unobtainable at certain times of the year.

My own grandmother, stooped by osteoporosis, became an invalid late in life, despite the fact that her doctors told her, even then, she needed to walk every day. She obstinately refused. She lived a long life, but her last thirty years were severely limited. By comparison, my mother, at a sprightly eighty, considers it her job to go to the gym every day. She's religious about it. I doubt my grandmother ever saw the inside of a gym.

I'm now in my late fifties, the same age my grandmother was when she became a widow and began her long physical slide. As a child, I thought of her as a decrepit old woman. I'm not like her in that way. I walk a couple of miles a day, ride my horse several times a week, and engage in almost daily bouts of vigorous gardening, kicked up by an occasional leap out of an airplane at 10,000 feet. My grandmother would be appalled!

Easy Approaches

A program of diet, exercise, and the right herbs and supplements can hand you long life on a platter. Not only can they reduce the symptoms of your perimenopause, they can work as well as hormone replacement, maybe even better in some cases. Certainly, diet and exercise can offer you protection against the serious and life-threatening diseases associated with aging. It's your choice. The upcoming chapters will help you decide what's best for you.

Great Sex after Fifty

Loss of interest in sex is common during perimenopause and after, and it's of great concern to many women. Any number of factors can influence a woman's sex drive at any time in her life, but in perimenopause and menopause, declining hormones can be a factor.

This is one part of menopause where declining estrogen levels may play an important role and where natural hormone replacement may be particularly helpful. In fact, testosterone is the hormone of desire in both men and women, and since testosterone levels sometimes drop as menopause approaches, it is possible they can affect sexual desire. If tests show that your testosterone or dehydroepiandrosterone (DHEA) levels are low, supplemental testosterone may help bring your libido back.

Estrogen plays a role. Dr. Christiane Northrup says declining levels of estradiol and progesterone also affect sexual arousal, sensitivity to touch, and orgasm because these hormones increase the flow of blood to sexually sensitive areas. Lower estrogen levels can also lead to thinning of vaginal tissue and a loss of lubrication, making intercourse uncomfortable. Low estrogen can also be responsible for a thinning of the urethral walls, which may be responsible for the minor urinary incontinence that can take place if you sneeze, cough, or laugh.

Progesterone has its place. Progesterone is also important in the sex equation. It has not been as well studied as estrogen and testosterone, but it has been shown to maintain sexual desire and keep it from fading. Since progesterone helps make estrogen and testosterone, sufficient levels of progesterone will help keep the entire hormonal trio functioning for sexual pleasure.

Among many other things, natural hormone replacement can help keep your libido active. This benefit should be part of your deliberations when you decide whether or not to take any hormone replacement. You'll find more information to help you make that decision in Chapter 11.

CHAPTER 6

POSTMENOPAUSE: A WOMAN'S NEEDS

In clinical terms, you have reached menopause when you have not had a menstrual period for twelve months. The average age for menopause for an American woman is fifty-two, but certain factors can affect the onset of full menopause. Menopause generally follows a perimenopause that can last as long as ten years, or it may come suddenly as a result of surgery, radiation therapy, or autoimmune disease. Smoking and some types of medications can also trigger early menopause.

Some experts theorize that the high levels of xenoestrogens in our environment (see Chapter 2) are actually causing women to reach *menarche* (the onset of menstruation) early and to reach menopause prematurely, as well.

What Happens in Menopause

When you reach menopause, your ovaries stop producing eggs and there is no possibility of further pregnancy. However, just because your ovaries have stopped producing eggs—and estrogen—doesn't mean you have no more estrogen. In theory, your adrenal glands will provide you with the estrogen you need. Your fat cells and your uterus also produce estrogen and, in theory, your liver processes and packages the hormones in conjunction with thyroid hormones. Notice, I said, "in theory."

Lorna Vanderhaeghe explains the problem elegantly in *An A-Z Woman's Guide to Vibrant Health*: "What makes the difference between a woman who has no symptoms at menopause and a woman who suffers with a multitude of symptoms? Women with exhausted adrenals, low levels of thyroid hormones, and a congested liver will have terrible menopause symptoms compared to women with a healthy liver, thyroid, and adrenals."

Adrenal Exhaustion

Since vast numbers of women approaching menopause are highly stressed, leading to adrenal exhaustion, and have low thyroid function, as well, it's not surprising that their symptoms grow worse as full menopause approaches. Symptoms of adrenal exhaustion are similar to those experienced by many women with low thyroid levels or in perimenopause.

Adrenal function self-test. An easy self-test can be done if you have a blood-pressure monitor and someone to take your blood pressure:

1. Lie quietly on your back for at least five minutes.

2. Record your blood pressure.

3. Sit up quickly, and take your blood pressure again.

4. Stand up quickly, and take it again.

In people with normal adrenal function, the blood pressure will rise between 4 and 10 points with each measurement. If your blood pressure drops for either of the last two measurements, it's a strong sign that your adrenal glands are exhausted.

Too Much Estrogen

Too much estrogen has its downside after menopause, as well. Excess estrogen in your system can lead to endometrial hyperplasia (excessive growth of the uterine lining) and uterine fibroid tumors. Estrogen dominance is caused when there is insufficient progesterone to balance the ever-changing amounts of estrogen your system is making.

Plummeting Testosterone

By the time a women reaches menopause, her testosterone levels have also dropped—by approximately 50 percent. This leads to depression, fatigue, irritability, joint pain, loss of interest in sex, loss of muscle development, thin and dry skin, and osteoporosis. In *The HRT Solution*, Marla Ahlgrimm suggests that testosterone replacement in menopause "can re-ignite a woman's libido, restore a youthful level of energy, rejuvenate her, and renew her enthusiasm." And we know that testosterone plays a key role in bone health and may help prevent osteoporosis.

Happy Outcome

Many women fear that the symptoms of perimenopause will last forever. Happily, no! Although the symptoms may be intense for as long as ten years, Dr. Christiane Northrup aptly describes the process of adapting to a new hormonal structure. "In this culture, the symptoms of perimenopause, in a natural transition, last anywhere from five to ten years, with a gradual *crescendo* in the beginning, a peak as the women approaches the midpoint of the transition, and a gradual *decrescendo* as the body learns to live in harmony with its new hormonal support system."

Timeline

Perimenopause. Irregular periods, mood swings, and other symptoms may take place as many as ten years before the last menstrual period.

Menopause. Twelve months after the last menstrual period, a woman is in full menopause. Some perimenopausal symptoms will continue for as long as five years after menopause.

The Big Risks

Menopause means an increased risk of heart disease, osteoporosis, and Alzheimer's disease. It's serious, and it's important. Hot flashes, mood swings, and irritability may be the subject of jokes. They're not fun for you, but you can probably laugh at yourself from time to time.

No one laughs at heart disease, osteoporosis, or Alzheimer's disease. This is when we start to get serious about finding ways to maintain the hormonal protection we had against these diseases when we were younger. Now is the time you need estrogen. And if your adrenals, your fat cells, and your uterus aren't producing enough, you're at risk of the Big Four: heart disease, cancer, osteoporosis, and Alzheimer's disease.

Heart Disease

Heart disease was once considered to be a man's disease, but not anymore. We know better now. Heart disease is the leading cause of death in menopausal women. Although younger women have a far lower risk of heart disease than men, by the time a woman reaches menopause, her risk is equal to a man's. One in ten American women aged forty-five to sixty-four has some form of heart disease, and this number increases to one in four for women over sixty-five.

A woman's annual risk of dying from heart disease is more than double her risk of dying from all cancers combined. Women are twice as likely as men to suffer heart attacks, and they are more at risk for second heart attacks and more susceptible to sudden death from heart attack.

Subtle symptoms. Part of the problem is that the symptoms of heart attack in women are much more subtle than those found in men. For example:

- Shortness of breath, often without chest pain of any kind

- Flu-like symptoms—specifically nausea, clammi-ness, or cold sweats

- Unexplained fatigue, weakness, or dizziness

- Pain in the chest, upper back, shoulders, neck, or jaw

- Feelings of anxiety, loss of appetite, discomfort

Women are less likely to experience the chest-crushing pain and numbness in the left arm that characterize a heart attack in men. That's why doctors often misdiagnose a woman who has had a heart attack.

The other part of the problem is the obvious one: As a woman ages, hormone production is reduced and the loss of the protective effect of female hormones increases her risk. As estrogen levels go down, the risk of heart disease goes up.

Estrogen helps. Appropriate estrogen levels have been shown to:

- Increase HDL, or "good" cholesterol

- Lower levels of fibrinogen, the substance that causes blood clotting

- Lower blood pressure and improve elasticity of blood vessels

- Lower blood levels of homocysteine, a marker for heart disease

The latest research suggests that estrogen is not alone among hormones in protecting against heart disease. Testosterone, dehydroepiandroster - one (DHEA), and progesterone also appear to play a role in protecting your heart. (See Chapter 11 for a detailed explanation of natural hormone replace-ment therapy [HRT].)

Cancer
We know that cancer is not solely the concern of

postmenopausal women. People of all ages get cancer. In fact, the lifetime risk of any individual getting some form of cancer is one in three. The average American woman has a 13.2 percent chance of developing breast cancer sometime in her life, according to the National Cancer Institute. The average American woman between the ages of sixty and sixty-nine (postmenopausal) has a 1 in 26 chance of getting breast cancer. While those numbers are daunting, there are many things you can do to reduce your risk.

Hormone-related cancers. After menopause, you are more vulnerable to hormone-related cancer, such as breast, ovarian, uterine, and cervical cancers. It's not surprising that estrogen—the right kind of estrogen—and progesterone play an important role in preventing all these types of cancer. Scientists know that the incidence of breast cancer increases as a woman enters her forties. Why? Because declining progesterone levels and fluctuating estrogen levels promote unopposed estrogen and can promote the wild cell growth seen in breast cancer and other hormone-related cancers.

> **Unopposed Estrogen**
> *Estrogen acting without the balancing and protective effects of progesterone.*

Studies show that progesterone plays a role in preventing uterine cancer and possibly breast cancer, as well. Progesterone endorses the "key and lock" combination with estrogen that helps estrogen work for you. Progesterone has also been shown to increase the growth of natural killer (NK) cells, a type of white blood cells that is your body's first line of defense against the growth of all types of cancer cells.

Animal studies have shown that estrogen taken in combination with progesterone substantially reduces the incidence of certain types of cancer. In *The HRT Solution*, Marla Ahlgrimm says, "This suggests if you provide estrogen and progesterone together, in the way they occur naturally in the body, the development of cancer may be less likely. In this way, science is showing us that it may not be the hormones themselves, but taking overdoses of individual hormones that increases the cancer risk."

Eating a diet high in antioxidant vegetables and fruits and rich in whole grains and healthy fats (see Chapter 7) will go a long way toward protecting you against these dreaded cancers. Nevertheless, cancer can strike seemingly without reason. Keeping yourself in good overall health, exercising regularly, and limiting your exposure to chemicals and toxins will help to protect you.

If you smoke, please, please, please, do everything you can to quit. Smoking dramatically increases your risk of several types of cancer. Some studies link cancer with emotional stress and negative thinking. The better you can manage your stress and intentionally create positive thought, the more protection you'll have.

Osteoporosis

Brittle bones, dowager's hump, and fear of fracture are the primary reasons that many postmeno-pausal women choose to curtail their physical activity. Women are four times more likely to get osteoporosis than men, suggesting a hormonal component in the progress of this disease.

The National Osteoporosis Foundation estimates that 10 million Americans have osteoporosis and another 34 million have osteopenia, or low bone density. The risk of osteoporosis is highest among non-Hispanic white and Asian women. Falling estrogen levels can cause bones to become thin and brittle, but increased estrogen levels alone won't reverse the loss of bone density.

In *Natural Woman, Natural Menopause*, Dr. Marcus Laux says estrogen replacement can slow bone loss, but progesterone replacement can actually help build bone mass. Laux also links testosterone and DHEA to increased bone mass. The best way to learn about the health of your bones is to have a bone-density scan.

Plastic bones. Conventional medicine has a love affair with a much-promoted anti-osteoporosis drug called Fosamax. While research shows that it helps build bone mass, the bone it makes is not the same as natural bone; it's actually more susceptible to fracture. Laux says, "Once you start (Fosamax), you shouldn't stop. And the bone-mineral crystal that is formed is immovable. This brings up innumerable concerns about the bone's ability to function naturally or even heal itself." Laux's recommendation about Fosamax: "Approach with flashing red caution lights."

For stronger bones. Calcium alone is not enough. While calcium is important for bone rigidity (the recommended daily intake for postmenopausal women is 1,500 milligrams), magnesium, vitamin D, vitamin K, boron, manganese, and phosphorus also play important roles. You need all of them. For more information on these, see Chapter 9.

Exercise is not optional. Weight-bearing exercise is essential for strong bones; the earlier in life, the better. Recent studies show that girls who were physically active as teens had a lower chance of osteoporosis as they aged. But it's never too late to start. See Chapter 8 for a complete discussion of exercise.

Alzheimer's Disease

Partly because women live longer than men, we experience about double the risk of Alzheimer's disease, but it's also certain that estrogen plays a part in our increased risk. Estrogen influences language skills, mood, attention, and a number of other functions, in addition to memory.

There are estrogen receptors or docking sites

in several areas of the brain, including those that affect memory. Estrogen boosts the production of acetylcholine, a key brain chemical that helps transmit nerve impulses across the tiny gaps between nerve cells. Estrogen may raise the levels of certain brain chemicals, including noradrenaline (mood and other autonomic functions), serotonin (mood), and dopamine (motor coordination). Estrogen also helps nerves communicate better with one another.

Estrogen Receptors

The part of a cell that allows it to recognize estrogen. Estrogen can be thought of as a "key" and the receptor as a "lock"; so, estrogen opens the lock and allows the function to be performed.

Premarin does not protect your brain. The Women's Health Initiative had a component showing that synthetic or equine-based hormone replacement did not protect against Alzheimer's disease and, in fact, substantially increased the risk of dementia in older women. That study used equine-based estrogen and synthetic progesterone. However, there has been no research indicating whether bioidentical hormones might produce a different result. For more information on bioidentical hormones, see Chapter 11.

Other studies have suggested the opposite. Several studies show that women taking various combinations of HRT score better on memory and learning and have a slower decline in mental function than those not taking HRT. Two studies show that women who took HRT had a reduced risk of Alzheimer's disease. In one, the risk was lower by 60 percent. Bottom line: The jury is still out on estrogen and Alzheimer's disease.

CHAPTER 7

A SUITABLE DIET

You are what you eat! In *Get Off the Menopause Roller Coaster*, Dr. Shari Lieberman says diet is your best hormone replacement therapy (HRT). That's because dozens of plant-based hormones, called "phytohormones" or "phytoestrogens," have been shown to be effective in addressing a variety of perimenopausal symptoms. In fact, a well-balanced diet is the key to your health at any time in your life. Dozens of studies prove—yes, *prove*—that the people who eat the most fruits, veggies, whole grains, and legumes (dried beans and peas) have a lower risk of almost every type of cancer and a vastly reduced risk of heart disease and other age-related diseases.

Eat Your Veggies

Plant foods are the most powerful tools in your hormone-balancing nutrition arsenal. Multivitamins are good, too, but think of them as an insurance policy. Nothing can replace the complex combination of intertwined and interdependent nutrients you find in just one bite of broccoli or a single segment of an orange.

Consider a half-cup serving of the lowly broccoli stalk that has just 21 calories. It has:

- 1,082 mg of heart-protective, eyesight-preserving vitamin A.

- A respectable amount of bone-preserving calcium.

- An equally respectable amount of the anti - oxidant vitamin C.

- Isothiocyanates, plant compounds that have been clinically proven to protect against several types of cancer, including prostate and lung cancers.

- Indole-3 carbinol and sulforaphane, which protect against breast cancer.

- A respectable amount of weight-loss-inducing fiber.

So, what's not to love about broccoli?

Eat Colorful Foods

All types of foods have their own unique blends of healthy nutrients, so make your diet colorful and varied for maximum general health. Whatever the U.S. Department of Agriculture's (USDA's) latest food pyramid says, fresh fruits and vegetables need to be the core ingredients of everyone's diet. You've no doubt been encouraged to eat five servings of fruits and vegetables a day, but you may not know that the average American eats less than three servings a day. You may not know that five-a-day should be a *minimum*. We should be aiming for seven or nine servings a day or more. The more, the better! No one ever got fat on fruits and vegetables, but millions of people have gotten healthier. It's not as difficult as it sounds.

Get Ten a Day

Have a serving of fruit with your morning cereal or a sliced tomato with your eggs. A salad for lunch—two cups with lots of veggies added in, equals four servings. Wow! You're already up to five servings, and it's only lunchtime! Stir some fruit into your afternoon yogurt for a healthy snack, or spread some cream cheese on a few celery sticks. For dinner have another good-sized salad (at least a cup and a half) and a hefty serving of fresh veggies as a side dish. That's ten servings—painlessly.

Plant Power

This type of eating is not only healthy in general, it has specific benefits for those of us who are journeying through perimenopause and menopause in particular. Dr. Marcus Laux calls plants "master biochemists." That's because they have learned, through the process of evolution, to protect themselves from viruses, bacteria, predators, and even potentially harmful sunlight.

What's important to women as we enter menopause is that plants also have an endocrine system remarkably similar to ours. Plant hormones direct the operations in their own systems and produce their own forms of estrogen and progesterone, called phytohormones, which regulate growth and maturation much like our hormonal structure does. Plenty of research shows that women who eat large quantities of wholesome vegetables, fruits, whole grains, and legumes have more balanced hormonal systems. These plant hormones, when consumed by humans, are extraordinarily effective in combating menopause-related symptoms and in many cases can be an alternative to any form of hormone replacement, whether via herbs and supplements or prescription medications.

You've no doubt heard that Asian women do not experience perimenopausal and menopausal symptoms as Western women do. That's probably because the Asian lifestyle and diet are vastly different from those of the average Westerner. Asians eat huge quantities of vegetables and relatively small amounts of protein. They also eat soy products, such as *miso* and *tofu*, almost as a staple food. Researchers who took a deeper look at the contrast between cultures concluded that the Asian plant-based diet, especially its soy consumption, was providing a natural food-based HRT for women as they entered their menopausal years, allowing them to seamlessly weather hormonal fluctuations by simply eating the right foods.

Eat Right—Protect Your Breasts

Ample research shows that these phytohormones not only relieve perimenopausal discomforts such as hot flashes, but they are also protective against much more serious conditions such as breast cancer. Phytoestrogens are similar in structure to estriol—the form of estrogen that is most desirable during your menopausal years. They help neutralize the effects of estradiol, the form of estrogen least desirable at this time. They also help protect breast tissue against environmental toxins such as pesticides and air pollution. Phytohormones are literally the keys that fit in the estrogen-receptor site "locks," preventing disease, particularly breast cancer, from taking hold. They also promote a healthy liver, and since the liver uses phytoestrogens extensively in its proper function, a storehouse of phytoestrogens means there will be more healthy estriol in your body.

Getting phytohormones into your body does not mean shoveling in pound after pound of tasteless soybeans. It's as simple as eating a half-cup serving of phytoestrogen-rich foods each day. That can include soy products (there are delicious new soy-nut snacks on the market), chick peas (garbanzo beans), and any of the dozens of soy-based burgers and meat-replacement products on the market. Cruciferous vegetables such as broccoli, cauliflower, and cabbage are also excellent sources of phytohormones. Experts say that just these wonder foods alone may be enough to keep perimeno - pausal symptoms at bay.

The Five-Pound-a-Year Menace

Perhaps one of the worst effects of this hormonal roller coaster is the weight gain that frequently accompanies menopause. Take heart. It does not have to be that way. Fluctuating hormones cause food cravings, make our bodies hold on to the fat that's already there, and accumulate fat in places we never had it before. Thunder thighs and pear- and apple-shaped bodies aren't inevitable. You can avoid menopausal weight gain by keeping your hormones balanced and eating a sensible diet rich in vegetables, fruits, whole grains, lean meats, fish, and healthy fats.

Good Fat Gets a Good Rep

Fat has gotten a bad reputation in recent years, and it's totally undeserved. We must have healthy fats to survive. The hard part is sorting out the good fats from the bad fats. Let's make it as easy as possible. These foods qualify as good fats: fatty cold-water fish such as salmon, tuna, mackerel, and shrimp; and the oils of virtually all kinds of vegetables, including soy, olive, flaxseed, safflower, and sunflower. These bad fats are best to avoid: margarine, any fat that stays solid at room temperature (such as Crisco); and excessive amounts of fatty meats.

Why are fish and olive oil good for you and margarine and Crisco bad? Good fats are sources of essential fatty acids, which have been study-proven to actually protect your heart and promote cardiovascular health, strengthen your immune system, and prevent everything from colds and flu to cancer. They're also essential to a healthy menopause, since eating a balance of fatty acids can balance hormones, addressing problematic hot flashes, irritability, depression, and headaches. Bad fats are packed with saturated fat and even polyunsaturated fat that actually promote the building of layers of plaque in your arteries, leading to heart disease and dramatically increasing your risk of heart attack and stroke.

Getting the right fats is not as difficult as it might sound. Simply substituting olive oil for bottled salad dressings and sprinkling a teaspoon of ground flaxseed on your salad will go a long way toward bringing you into the healthy fat category. If you substitute broiled salmon for that fatty steak or a tuna-salad sandwich for that greasy burger even once a week, you'll be doing your heart and your health a favor.

Make a Commitment to the Basics

Here are a few basic rules that will not only ease your menopause, but also keep you healthy whether you've decided to live to be eighty, ninety, or 110!

1. **Five a day without fail.** Commit yourself completely to getting at least five servings of fruits and vegetables a day—no exceptions— even if it means you're chowing down on carrot sticks at 11:59 P.M.

2. **Opt for natural.** Eat as many fresh foods as possible. If you can't always get fresh veggies, frozen is next best. Canned veggies have most of their nutrients cooked out.

3. **Eat the rainbow.** The more colorful the foods you eat, the more nutrients they contain. It's nature's way of attracting your eyes to the things that are best for you. Think red juicy tomatoes, crisp orange carrots, lush green broccoli, and so on.

4. **Go brown.** Ditch the white bread, white rice, and any baked goods made with white flour. They have few nutrients and almost no fiber. Whole grains are rich sources of magnesium, zinc, chromium, B vitamins, and fiber. Plus they're much more satisfying, so you'll eat less with a bigger vitamin bang for your buck.

5. **Lose the junk food.** Potato chips, tortilla chips, Ho-Ho's, Twinkies, and Ding Dongs, or whatever they call them, are terrible for your health, your heart, and your waistline. No two ways about it. They're an evil brew of bad fats and empty calories. If you can't give up the

crackle and crunch, go for a (small) handful of nuts, a little popcorn, or a few pretzels. To deal with the sweet tooth, have a cup of homemade cocoa made with skim milk and stevia, a healthy no-calorie sweetener. If you really get the chocolate urge, satisfy yourself with a single piece of high-quality dark chocolate.

6. **Choose white (meat).** Eat red meat in moderation, and make poultry, wild-caught fish, and legumes the centerpieces of your protein menu. Try to keep your red-meat meals to three or four a week. Have a vegetarian dinner at least once a week.

7. **Go light on dairy.** Many milk products and cheeses are high in calories and high in fat. Use skim milk, keep your cheese consumption moderate, and enjoy nonfat yogurt.

8. **Say no to fried foods.** Those French fries really pile on the pounds. Donuts are death to your arteries. Instead of frying, steam, bake, broil, or poach your foods. You can make delicious—and healthy—oven fries by slicing a couple of antioxidant-rich Russet potatoes with just a couple of tablespoons of healthy olive oil and a liberal dose of spices and sliding them under the broiler for a few minutes.

9. **Switch to seed oils.** Stop using bottled salad dressings. Never buy Crisco. Make your stir-fry with olive oil and a few drops of tasty sesame-seed oil. Buy extra-virgin olive oil for the best health benefits, and make all your oils organic if possible. Safflower, canola, and walnut oils are excellent for baking or other types of cooking where the strong flavor of olive oil isn't desirable.

10. **Everything in moderation.** Be moderate in your intake of these foods:

- **Caffeine, soft drinks (including diet), and refined sugar.** They leech minerals from your bones, and sugar adds calories with no food value.

- **Salt.** Most table salt is highly refined. Try sea salt instead, which contains a wealth of minerals.

- **Alcohol.** Keep your intake to two drinks a day or less, since alcohol has been known to knock your hormones out of whack. Red wine is best because it contains a wealth of disease-fighting antioxidants and helps reduce the risk of heart disease.

11. **Never say die.** Don't think of this eating advice as a diet. We all know the first three letters of diet are d-i-e. Take it one day at a time. Don't deprive yourself. Enjoy life, eat to live, and give your body the best food you can.

Fall Off the Wagon, and Get Right Back On

If you find yourself being consumed by the McDonald's monster, give in once in a while, but don't give in to guilt. None of us wants those five-pound-a-year blues, so be moderate, but keep in mind what five pounds a year means by the time you're ninety-nine! Recognize that there may be occasional cravings and deal with them and yourself gently; then, get back on track. If you must eat that cinnamon roll, treat yourself to a nice long walk afterward. You'll burn off the calories and double your pleasure. You really can't go wrong with this simple eating plan.

CHAPTER 8

THE BEST EXERCISE

Exercise! Most of us groan at the sound of the word. We think of bulging spandex, sweat-saturated gyms, and guys with greased muscles and overdeveloped egos. Who wants that? Exercise can be fun. In fact, it *must be* fun or you won't keep it up. So, here's the key to your entire program: Pick something you really love to do. For some of us, that means getting involved in a group activity. For others, it means blessed solitude. For still others, it means a mix of the two.

Miracle Drug

Exercise is the miracle drug that can:

- Decrease your risk of breast cancer by 50 percent
- Protect you against heart disease by lowering cholesterol and blood pressure
- Grant you long life
- Improve your immune system and overcome anemia
- Improve your memory
- Increase bone density and strength
- Make your skin look younger

Exercise Stimulates Hormones

Most of us are familiar with these positive effects of exercise, but most of us are probably unaware that exercise can have a positive effect on hormones, too. Exercise has been shown to increase testosterone levels in women. One study reported that blood levels of estrogen, testosterone, and growth hormone were significantly higher in women aged nineteen to sixty-nine after forty minutes of either endurance or resistance exercise when compared to a control group that performed no exercise. Even the older women produced more anti-aging hormones. The study concluded that "an acute bout of exercise can increase concentrations of anabolic hormones in females across a wide age range." All this is a great incentive to get moving.

Weight-Bearing Exercise

Here is your new mantra: weight-bearing exercise. It keeps your bones strong. It's great for your heart. People who exercise live longer—it's as simple as that. Plus it settles your mind. Weight-bearing exercise is simple: It's any kind of exercise where you're on your feet.

The most popular weight-bearing exercise is walking. It's been study-proven to offer tremendous protection against heart disease, even if you walk only twenty minutes a day. And it's inexpensive. All you need is a good pair of walking shoes. Is twenty minutes more than you can handle? Take a ten-minute walk before lunch and another just before dinner. If you're a morning person, there are few better ways to start the day than to make a brisk sunrise walk part of your daily schedule.

Take the pledge. If walking isn't your "thing," try jogging, tennis, squash, cycling, volleyball, or aerobics. Remember, you've got to love it or you won't do it, so pick one, or better yet, two or three, activities you really enjoy. Make your pledge now: Do weight-bearing exercise every day.

Keep it simple. Remember, this plan is all about simplicity, so keep your exercise simple. Go for a walk every day. Enjoy the birds singing, smell the flowers, greet your neighbors. Better yet, strap on a pair of two-pound wrist weights, and swing your arms vigorously as you walk to get in your upper-body strength-training workout. Try a little shadow boxing, just for fun.

10,000 steps. Clip a pedometer to your belt, and see how many steps you take in a day. The goal is 10,000 steps (about four miles). You'll be surprised by how many steps you take walking around your office, in and out of the supermarket, chasing kids up and down the stairs, hauling laundry, and vacuuming the living room.

Look for extras. Do you love gardening? An hour of vigorous gardening can burn as many as 480 calories! Are you into home improvement? Hauling lumber, pounding nails, and climbing into the rafters count as weight-bearing exercise and strength training. If you love tennis, by all means, play. If your kids or grandkids are playing Frisbee in the yard, join them. Go for a hike. Run in your local fun run. Join a mall-walkers group, especially if you live in a place where weather might be an excuse or where your safety is an issue. (Hint: Leave your credit cards at home!) The possibilities are endless. It's not important what you do, it's just important that you do it.

Can't Seem to Squeeze in Time for a Walk?

You've heard all this before. It truly is painless.

- Take the stairs instead of the elevator.

- Park as far away from the mall entrance as possible.

- Jog in place while you're talking on the phone.

- Get a large dog. He'll insist that you walk him twice daily.

- Get your spouse to take a walk with you after dinner rather than plunking down in front of the TV.

- If all else fails, get one of those little jogging trampolines, and do a workout (with hand weights) while you watch the evening news.

Too Tired to Get Moving?

Make a firm, unbreakable vow to yourself that you'll do it anyway for three weeks. You'll find that your energy levels will pump up so much that you'll wonder why you were ever so tired. Warning: Exercise is addictive. Aerobic exercise kicks in natural pain killers, morphine-like brain chemicals called endorphins, which are actually addictive. Your brain releases endorphins when you exercise, so you literally become addicted to the natural high you get. This is a positive addiction!

Am I Working Hard Enough?

Figure Your Target Heart Rate:

- Subtract your age from 220. This gives you your maximum heart rate.

- Multiply by 0.70.

- The result is your training target rate.

For example, if you're fifty-five years old, your maximum heart rate would be 165, and your training target rate would be 116. You'll get more aerobic activity if you go up to 80 percent of your maximum, but don't go beyond that unless you are a highly trained athlete.

To Measure Your Heart Rate:

- The moment you stop exercising, place the fingers of your left hand near the base of your throat. You'll feel your heartbeat.

- Count the number of beats in ten seconds.

- Multiply by 6.

- The total is your current heart rate.

Strength Training

Now, I'm asking you to take a second pledge: Do strength-training exercises at least three times a week. You don't have to develop bulging muscles or take on Venus Williams. All you need is a couple of hand weights and an exercise band or tubing resistance bands. They're inexpensive, and they're available wherever sporting goods are sold. It's a good idea to have varying weights and strengths so you can keep up the challenge as you build your strength. In a pinch, you can even use refilled water bottles for hand weights.

Use the exercise bands or tubing to strengthen legs and tone your "glutes" (buttocks). Three twenty-minute workouts a week will do the trick. It might be helpful to invest in a session or two with a professional trainer to learn a routine and to be certain you're doing the exercises correctly. As an alternative, check out a few videos from your local library so you can build a routine that works for you. You might even want to invest in a video once you find one you like.

Just Do It

It doesn't matter how you do it, just do it. Just twenty minutes a day will make a huge difference in your life. Do it for me, do it for your significant other, do it for your kids. Most of all, do it for yourself, and do it *every* day. You'll love yourself for it.

Beyond weight-bearing exercise, more and more research is showing the benefits of East-ern forms of exercise: *yoga, tai chi,* and *chi gong.* All of these are excellent for keeping your body flexible and improving balance and posture, two major ways to protect yourself against bone loss.

There's also a much more subtle aspect to these art forms. They utilize universal energy, called *prana* by the yogis and *chi* or *ki* by practitioners of *tai chi* and *chi gong.* Bringing this energy into your body through coordinated movement and breath makes your entire being feel and look awake, alert, youthful—and, most of all, relaxed. See Chapter 10 for more about these aspects of the Eastern disciplines. Look for a local class or buy a tape from a reputable teacher (see the Other Books and Resources section), and get an entirely new outlook on life.

CHAPTER 9

NATURAL HERBS AND SUPPLEMENTS

For many of us, diet and exercise just aren't enough to manage perimenopausal symptoms. And after menopause, issues of heart disease and cancer are most likely best addressed with vitamins, minerals, herbs, or other supplements.

Multivitamins

A good multivitamin will give you the foundation you need, not only for good nutrition, but also for general good health. In fact, in 2003 the *Journal of the American Medical Association (JAMA)*, a stalwart of mainstream medicine, recommended a daily multivitamin for everyone—adults and children. Why? Because even if you grow your own organic produce, it's impossible to know how many minerals your veggies can pull from our depleted soil.

Most of us buy whatever is available in the supermarket. Our food has been picked before it reached its peak nutritional quality, and transported for several days before it gets to the grocer's shelves, losing nutrients every step of the way. So, a multivitamin has become an essential part of health. It's important to find a good quality multivitamin that your body can use.

How to Tell What's Good

Look for a product that is natural, simply because it will not contain artificial coloring, preservatives, sugar, starch, coal tar, and other additives. Dr. Shari Lieberman recommends the ingredients in Table

9.1 as the basic amounts for a day's dosage of a good multivitamin/mineral.

TABLE 9.1. A GOOD MULTIVITAMIN/ MINERAL SHOULD CONTAIN . . .	
VITAMINS	
Vitamin A	5,000–10,000 IU
Beta-carotene (precursor to vitamin A)	10,000–25,000 IU
Vitamin B complex	
Thiamine	50–100 mg
Riboflavin	50–100 mg
Niacin	50–100 mg
Vitamin B_6	50–100 mg
Folic acid	400–800 mcg
Vitamin B_{12}	50–100 mg
Biotin	10–50 mcg
Pantothenic acid	10–50 mg
Inositol	10–25 mg
Para-aminobenzoic acid (PABA)	10–25 mg
Vitamin C	500–1,000 mg
Vitamin D	400–800 IU
Vitamin E	200–600 IU
Minerals	
Boron	1–3 mg
Calcium	1,500 mg
Chromium	50–200 mcg
Copper	0.5–2 mg
Iodine	50–150 mcg
Magnesium	250–500 mg
Manganese	5–15 mg
Selenium	50–200 mcg
Zinc	15–50 mg

You may not find a single product that contains these precise amounts, but look for something that comes as close as possible.

Supplements for Perimenopause and Menopause

These well-researched supplements can offer relief from the symptoms of perimenopause and menopause. They may also help prevent more serious illnesses related to declining progesterone and fluctuating estrogen.

Black Cohosh (Cimecifuga racemosa)

This is the gold standard for treating many symptoms of perimenopause and menopause. It's effective for large numbers of women, so try this one first. Black cohosh is extremely effective against hot flashes, the number-one complaint of women in perimenopause. It's also useful to combat fatigue, headaches, insomnia, irritability, mood swings, and night sweats. Black cohosh is one of the most widely studied herbs that addresses these symptoms and helps to stabilize blood pressure and relieve heart palpitations.

Dosage. Take two 20-mg capsules or tablets daily standardized to 1-mg terpene glycosides per 20-mg tablet.

Side effects. No adverse effects have ever been reported, although most scientific studies have limited use to six months. Remifemin is the brand used in many clinical trials on the effectiveness of black cohosh.

Soy Isoflavones

Soy is a rich source of plant estrogens that have a structure similar to that of human estrogen, and it affects the way estrogen is metabolized in your body without the negative side effects. Think of those lovely, slender Japanese women who eat soy every day in the form of *miso* soup and *tofu*, and who remain slim, remarkably free from breast cancer, and pass through menopause with barely a bead of sweat on their brows. Their language does not even have a word for hot flash! Recent British research shows that the isoflavones in soy may help prevent breast cancer while reducing the risk of heart disease and osteoporosis.

Dosage. At least 100 mg per day.

Side effects. More is not better. Excessive soy has its downside: Too much estrogen relative to other hormones can be as problematic as not having enough. If you are on kidney dialysis or if you have had a hormone-related cancer or are risk for one (for example, breast or ovarian cancer), talk to your doctor before taking soy isoflavones.

Vitex (Vitex agnus castus)

Also known as chasteberry, vitex has been used for centuries to help banish those vicious mood swings during perimenopause by balancing your estrogen and progesterone levels. It can also help relieve hot flashes. Vitex also supports normal menstrual function, so it can help relieve heavy and irregular periods, enhance skin health, and balance the function of the pituitary gland.

Dosage. Take 6–80 mg per day in capsule form or 40 drops of liquid extract.

Side effects. Vitex has, on rare occasion, been known to cause headaches, weight gain, nausea, and diarrhea. The side effects disappear quickly if you stop taking it.

Red Clover (Trifolium pratense)

This wonder herb, found in pastures everywhere, is a rich source of isoflavones, the same compounds found in soy. Isoflavones stimulate the ovaries to increase estrogen production—maximizing what you have even as perimenopause progresses. Red clover is very helpful in relieving hot flashes and it may help to relieve joint pain, but its true beauty is in the ability of the isoflavones to help protect you against heart disease and osteoporosis. Red clover may also be valuable in treating some types of non-hormonal cancers.

Dosage. Take 1–3 grams (g) daily.

Side effects. None known.

Coenzyme Q_{10} (CoQ$_{10}$)

CoQ_{10} is your body's energy catalyst. It is the beginning point of a chain of chemical reactions that creates the energy your cells need to function at optimal level. It's also a powerful antioxidant that gobbles up disease-causing free radicals. CoQ_{10} is particularly important in preventing heart disease and treating existing heart disease.

Dosage. The benchmark is about 1 mg per pound of body weight.

Side effects. Include mild gastrointestinal upset. If this occurs, reduce the dosage slightly.

L-Carnitine

This nutrient, which addresses a host of peri-menopausal and menopausal complaints, is found in meat and dairy products, but you probably need it even if you're not a vegetarian. L-carnitine is widely used to improve brain function and mental sharpness, assist in weight loss, and increase general energy levels. Because L-carnitine helps all cells to use their energy more efficiently, it also helps your body stay young. If that's not enough, L-carnitine helps keep blood fats (triglycerides) low and HDL or "good" cholesterol high—just where you want them to be.

Dosage. Take 500–4,000 mg daily, depending on your reason for using the supplement. Go toward the higher end for weight loss or if your doctor has told you that you have seriously high triglycerides. Dosages in the range of 500–2,000 mg are helpful in relieving the symptoms of premenstrual syndrome (PMS), and doses as low as 300 mg are helpful in combating depression and mood swings.

Side effects. In rare cases, it can cause increased blood pressure, faster heartbeats, fever, and diarrhea.

Dong Quai (Angelica sinensis)

This fragrant herb has been used in Asia for centuries to relieve hot flashes, mood swings, insomnia, night sweats, and headaches.

Dosage. Take one 200–mg capsule three times a day.

Side effects. Because it enhances estrogen, *dong quai* can intensify bleeding, so do not use this herb during your menstrual period if you have heavy bleeding.

Dehydroepiandrosterone (DHEA)

If your lab tests have shown that your DHEA levels are low, DHEA supplements may help to bring you back into balance and relieve stress. Your body converts DHEA into estrogen, progesterone, and testosterone.

Dosage. Usually, you need 5–50 mg, but the exact amount is dependent on your lab results, and you should take it under a doctor's supervision.

Side effects. Taking too much can make your hormones even more unbalanced, worsening symptoms.

Evening Primrose Oil (Oenothera biennis)

This seed oil is a good source of gamma-linolenic acid (GLA), which is derived from linoleic acid, an essential fatty acid from the omega-6 family. In your body, linoleic acid is converted into a hormone-like substance called "prostaglandin PGE-1," which works as an anti-inflammatory and acts as a blood thinner and blood-vessel dilator. Evening primrose oil is used for general health, for the irritability and mood swings associated with PMS, for perimeno-pause, and for menopause. It may also be effective against hot flashes. Note: Borage oil has many of the same effects.

Dosage. Take 1,300 mg daily.

Side effects. None known.

Supplements for Strong Bones

Osteoporosis is one of the greatest fears of aging women, for good reason. As many as 36 percent of older women with an osteoporotic hip fracture will die within a year. The following supplements will help keep bones strong.

Calcium

This bone-building mineral is essential for women of all ages, particularly those beyond menopause. It adds structure and rigidity to bones. Correct levels of calcium protect against high blood pressure and keep the heart beating regularly. If you have inadequate calcium intake, your body will take calcium from the bones to keep your heart strong. The calcium in dairy products has also been shown to help control weight.

Dosage. For perimenopausal and menopausal women, take 1,200–1,500 mg per day.

Side effects. None known at the recommended dosage.

Magnesium

An important element of bone health, magnesium helps bones absorb calcium. Approximately 50 percent of the body's magnesium stores is found in the bones, but this mineral is essential to more than 300 biochemical reactions in the body. It helps maintain normal muscle and nerve function, keeps heart rhythm steady, supports a healthy immune system, and keeps bones strong. Magnesium also helps regulate blood-sugar levels and promotes normal blood pressure.

Dosage. At least 400 mg of magnesium a day. Many experts recommend 600 mg.

Side effects. None known at the recommended dosage.

Vitamin D$_3$

Essential to calcium absorption and bone mineralization, Vitamin D$_3$ has been shown to slow the rate of bone loss.

Dosage. Take 400–800 IU daily.

Side effects. None known at the recommended dosage.

Vitamin K

This vitamin helps to maintain osteocalcin, a hormone necessary for bone-building, and hold calcium in the bones.

Dosage. Take 100 mcg daily.

Side effects. Vitamin K is a known blood thinner, so it helps to keep blood from clotting and prevent plaque buildup in the arteries. It may make your blood too thin if you are also taking a prescription blood thinner such as Coumadin.

Boron

This trace mineral is essential for calcium metabolism. It helps hold calcium and magnesium in the bones. Some researchers think it has estrogen-like effects; others think it has testosterone-like effects.

Dosage. Up to 3 mg.

Side effects. None known at the recommended dosage.

Supplements to Prevent Heart Disease

Since heart disease is the number-one killer of postmenopausal women, it's time to protect your cardiovascular system *now!*

Garlic (Allium sativum)

Common household garlic is one of the most potent herb tonics known—meaning that it works for a wide variety of conditions. Garlic protects your heart by preventing the formation of artery-clogging plaque, and it keeps your cholesterol levels in healthy ranges. So, all women past menopause and any women at risk for heart disease should take garlic every day.

Recent research shows that garlic is also protective against several types of cancer, and it may help prevent the complications associated with type 2 diabetes, including kidney failure, blindness, and slow wound-healing. Garlic also helps neutralize the effects of high-fat meals and improves immune-system function. Many people object to the odor of garlic, so if you're squeamish about adding large quantities of it to your food, take it in the deodorized form in capsules.

Dosage. Take 600–1,200 mg per day.

Side effects. None known (except perhaps social ostracism).

Policosanol

This derivative of beeswax has been clinically proven effective against high cholesterol, reducing your risk of heart disease and stroke. Policosanol helps bring cholesterol to normal levels— reducing it by 25 to 30 percent in six months or less. It also helps keep clots from forming, further protecting you from heart attacks and strokes.

Dosage. Take 10–15 mg at night.

Side effects. None known.

Supplements for Depression and Brain Function

Approximately 12 percent of American women suffer from clinical depression. Hundreds of thousands more have subclinical depression that is likely to worsen as they age. Moreover, declining memory is a problem for most elderly people, and more so for women who have taken equine-based HRT.

The following supplements have been scientifically validated for the treatment of depression and memory loss.

Ginkgo (Ginkgo biloba)

This powerful antioxidant came into the spotlight a few years ago with scientific research that showed it may be helpful in treating Alzheimer's disease, in addition to its already known heart-protective properties. Since then, ginkgo has become an enormously powerful remedy for short- and long-term memory loss and mental confusion. It is helpful for all sorts of memory problems, fatigue, and depression.

Dosage. Take up to 240 mg daily, and be sure you get a brand standardized to 24 percent *Ginkgo biloba* content.

Side effects. Acts as a blood thinner, so use with caution if taking other blood thinners, such as Coumadin or aspirin, or if you are planning surgery.

Kava Kava (Piper methysticum)

Kava kava provides a relaxed feeling coupled with mental sharpness. It gives you the relaxation you might get with a glass of wine and the mental sharpness you get with a cup of coffee, with none of the harmful side effects of either. Kava kava is great for stress relief and to help you sleep. It's also helpful to relieve stiff and achy joints. Research shows it is helpful in relieving the symptoms of menopause, as well.

Dosage. Take up to 60–75 mg of kavalactones two to four times daily. Look for a brand that is standardized to 30 percent kavalactones, and then multiply by the percent to get your dosage. For example, 200 mg of 30 percent kavalactones yields 60 mg.

Side effects. Do not use if you have impaired liver function. Do not mix with alcohol or other sedatives. Use caution when driving. Do not take on a regular basis for more than three months at a time.

SAM-e

In 95 percent of clinical studies, S-adenosylmethionine (SAM-e) was proven to be at least as effective as prescription antidepressants, helping 60 to 70 percent of depressed patients feel better—fast. And it works much faster—in five to ten days, as opposed to about a month for the prescription mood-enhancers.

Dosage. Take 200 mg once or twice daily between meals, increasing gradually to a maximum of 1,600 mg daily.

Side effects. Do not take SAM-e if you are tak - ing prescription antidepressants. SAM-e can trigger manic episodes in people with bipolar disorder.

Trimethylglycine (TMG)

Sometimes called the "poor man's SAM-e," tri - methylglycine (TMG), a.k.a. betaine, actually helps your body form the antidepressant SAM-e natur - ally—at a fraction of the cost! What's more, TMG lowers levels of artery-clogging homocysteine.

Dosage. Take 500–1,000 mg twice daily.

Side effects. None known at this dosage.

St. John's Wort

The latest research proves St. John's wort works wonderfully for people with mild to moderate depression—relieving it as well as prescription anti-depressants do but without the side effects. In fact, St. John's wort has been shown to *increase* sexual desire instead of dampening it. German research shows that it reduced depressive symptoms in nearly 70 percent of patients in just one week.

Dosage. Take 900 mg per day.

Side effects. Can cause stomach upset and nausea.

Note: There has been concern about serotonin buildup if St. John's wort is taken at the same time as prescription antidepressants. While there have been no documented cases of problems arising from this, it's wise to avoid St. John's wort if you're on prescription antidepressants.

The Best Weight-Control Supplements

There are hundreds of weight control products on the market. Many of them are useless. However, there is good, solid science behind the following supplements.

Alpha Lipoic Acid (ALA) and L-Carnitine

L-carnitine is a known fat burner and ALA helps burn glucose, leveling out blood-sugar swings and cravings. So, the two together have an extra impetus to help you lose weight. One Chinese study shows that women who added the supplement lost eleven pounds more than those who simply cut calories and increased exercise.

Dosage. Take 500 mg L-carnitine and 200 mg of ALA twice a day.

Side effects. None known at the recommended dosage.

L-Carnitine and Chromium

L-carnitine, a protein-like nutrient naturally produced by the liver and kidneys, and chromium, a
naturally occurring mineral, have long been used
to help with weight loss. Now, private laboratory
research in California suggests that the two to -
gether may help increase the fat-burning capacities
of the liver and help with weight loss. Scientists
have long known that chromium helps to make
your body's natural insulin supply work better,
keeping fat from being formed, and L-carnitine is
the only substance that can shovel fat into cellular
furnaces, called "mitochondria," to be burned for
energy.

Dosage. Take 1,000–1,200 mg of L-carnitine a day,
usually divided into doses taken morning and night,
and take 200–400 mcg of chromium a day. You may
find them in a high-powered combination that
adds hydroxycitric acid (HCA) into the mix.

Side effects. L-carnitine's side effects have been
enumerated above. Chromium is generally considered safe, although there have been animal studies
suggesting it may change DNA patterns in ham-
sters. It's unknown whether it affects human DNA.

Glutamine

This amino acid helps you produce calming brain
chemicals and is thought to help you feel full
longer. There is some research that suggests it
actually helps curb sugar and salt cravings by as
much as 50 percent.

Dosage. Take 1–2 g daily.

Side effects. None at the recommended dosage.

HCA (Garcinia cambogia)

Hydroxycitric acid (HCA) has been called the "jack-
of-all trades" of weight-loss supplements because
it targets many of the problem areas that cause

95 percent of all dieters to gain back what they've lost and more. It conserves and builds fat-burning lean muscle, curbs appetite, shuts down cravings, blocks fat production, and speeds up calorie-burning—all while giving you a great energy boost.

Dosage. Take HCA before each meal. Look for HCA in supplements manufactured by several different companies containing Citrimax or Citrin.

Side effects. None known at the recommended dosage.

Phase 2

This supplement, made from an extract of white kidney beans, helps prevent carbohydrate absorption by blocking amylase, the digestive enzyme that turns carbohydrates into sugar. Studies show that Phase 2 effectively neutralizes 66 percent of the carbohydrate calories you eat. Italian research shows taking two capsules before each meal typically triggers about a seven-pound weight loss in just thirty days—with no other changes in diet or exercise.

Dosage. Take twenty to thirty minutes before meals, according to manufacturer's instructions. Phase 2 is an ingredient in many products, including Phase 2 Carbohydrate Blocker by Source Naturals, Carb Intercept by Natrol, and Phase 2 by Vitamin Shoppe.

Side effects. None at the recommended dosage.

Whey Protein

This byproduct of milk can increase the production of lean-muscle tissue by 50 percent and enable you to burn 68 percent more body fat. Breakthrough research from Houston's Baylor University shows that a diet high in whey protein produced a weight loss of nearly twenty pounds in thirty weeks, and virtually eliminated the high blood sugars that are a precursor to diabetes. A study from Massachusetts Institute of Technology (MIT) says whey supplements help control appetite, probably because of whey's high content of mood-brightening tryptophan.

Dosage. Whey protein is usually sold as a powdered supplement and mixed with fruit juice or water. Follow the package instructions, and drink one or two whey smoothies a day.

Side effects. None known.

Supplements to Restore Sex Drive

Sex doesn't have to be a distant memory after menopause sets in. The following supplements have been documented to help increase sexual desire and function.

Maca (Lepidium meyenii)

If your sex drive has stalled, try this Peruvian root. It's been shown in clinical trials to increase sexual desire by 180 percent. Maca is a plant sterol that acts as a chemical trigger to signal your body to boost hormone production. Maca has been used traditionally for menstrual irregularities, hot flashes, fatigue, stress, and depression. Recent scientific studies suggest that it may help reverse low-thyroid conditions that are responsible for weight gain, fatigue, and low blood pressure.

Dosage. Take one 500-mg capsule with each meal.

Side effects. None known.

Damiana (Turnera diffusa, aphrodisiaca)

This South American herb is best known as an aphrodisiac; so, fasten your seat belt—it's time to enjoy sex again! Damiana is also a useful antidepressant, and its real beauty is that it can help break the cycle of depression/low sexual desire/depression. It's useful for headaches, and some studies suggest that damiana may have properties similar to testosterone.

Dosage. Take 3–4 g daily.

Side effects. None known, but if it doesn't relieve your symptoms in six weeks, try something else.

Ginkgo (Ginkgo biloba)

Best known for its memory-enhancing properties, ginkgo can also boost sex drive for people taking prescription antidepressants. Antidepressants such as Paxil and Prozac are known to reduce sexual desire in about half the patients who take them— both men and women. University of California (San Francisco) researchers found that just 120 mg of ginkgo extract a day restored sexual desire in 84 percent of the women who took it—without interfering with the effects of their prescription medications.

Dosage. Take up to 240 mg daily, and be sure you get a brand standardized to 24 percent ginkgo-flavonoid glycosides content.

Side effects. Acts as a blood thinner, so use with caution if taking other blood thinners, such as Coumadin or aspirin, or if you are planning surgery.

How to Use These Supplements

These remedies aren't like taking an aspirin and expecting your headache to disappear in a few minutes. If you decide to try any of them, give them several weeks to work. Many natural remedies, particularly herbs, take longer to work than phar-maceuticals because they are bringing about fundamental changes in your body, so be patient.

A word of caution: Many people believe that if a little bit of an herb or supplement is good for you, a handful is better. Don't do it! These are powerful medicines. They work. If the information accompanying the supplement you're considering says it has no side effects, that doesn't mean you can take unlimited quantities without a problem. Just as you wouldn't take a handful of blood-pressure pills or even aspirin, give herbs and supplements the same respect. Too much of anything can be harmful.

Remember, each human body is unique, so something that works for your best friend may not work for you. You need to do a little bit of experimenting to find the perfect combination for you.

(CHAPTER 10)

STRESS MANAGEMENT, MEDITATION, AND MORE

Menopause and perimenopause affect our entire being: body, mind, and spirit. Many of us are aware that our emotions directly affect our health. However, you may not know that emotions—positive and negative—affect every single cell and every hormone in your body. Dr. Christiane Northrup says that understanding this link between emotions and physical well-being is "the most powerful and empowering health-creating secret on earth." She says, "When all is said and done, it is your attitude, your beliefs, and your daily thought patterns that have the most profound effect on your health."

This is not meant to lay a guilt trip on you by suggesting that every hot flash or achy joint is karmic payback for some negative thought you had. But it has been scientifically documented that specific emotions are related to organs or systems in your body. Several studies show that breast cancer is connected to feelings of powerlessness and an inability to express emotions fully. Many other studies connect negative emotions and hostility to sudden death from a heart attack. And there are hundreds of studies that show that grief, separation, and loss of social support can impair immune function, opening the door to numerous diseases. This means that your health and your menopause are directly connected to the way you view the world.

The Stress Monster

Stress is a major component in all of our lives. It can't be eliminated. But we can choose how we address it. We've all seen those stress tests in magazines and scored ourselves, perhaps with some shock. However, stress is associated with positive events, as well as the ones we view as negative. Getting married, getting a big job promotion, or buying a house is recognized by your body in almost the same way as divorce, the serious illness of a loved one, or the loss of a job.

Fight or Flight

We've all heard of "fight-or-flight" syndrome. It sets off a very specific chain of physical responses when we are stressed. Imagine that you are driving home from work, relaxed and listening to some lovely classical music on your CD player. Suddenly, the driver to your right changes lanes without looking and without warning. Your body and mind kick into hyperdrive. Your heart begins to race. You probably say a choice word or two. Your vision becomes sharper, your reflexes speed up, and your brain becomes very alert as adrenaline is pumped through your system. You probably won't notice any physical sensation, but nonessential bodily systems, such as digesting your food, temporarily shut down so that your body's resources can be fully available to address the crisis.

Now is the time to decide whether to fight the threat or flee from it. This elegant response evolved in our prehistoric ancestors so they could escape the day-to-day physical threats to their existence. There could be many factors in the determination of whether to run away from the attacking saber-toothed tiger or to stand and fight. Regardless of the decision, we have the opportunity to preserve our lives thanks to our stress response.

You must decide in a split second how to deal with the guy who's cutting you off. There's little percentage in fighting him. You'd both probably get hurt—or worse. Therefore, you decide to flee. You warn him with your horn and swerve away, hoping there isn't a car in the lane to your left. The crisis ends well, and your heart rate slowly returns to normal, just as our ancestors' hearts did after they successfully evaded the saber-tooth tiger's attack.

But that's where the similarity ends. What we don't do that our ancestors did is to take some time to recover from the surge of adrenaline that caused a whole cascade of hormones to be released in our bodies. Our ancestors probably sat down, rested, discussed the threat, perhaps ate a meal—maybe even took a nap. But we "modern" folks continue the drive home, stop at the store, and are further stressed by waiting in a long line; get home, cook dinner, deal with wrangling kids, a mountain of laundry, and a spouse who is late. We pile these stressors on top of an impending deadline at work, concerns about our parents' health, a shortfall in our bank account, and on ... and on. It's all uncomfortably familiar. We don't give ourselves time to recover from stress and allow our systems to return to normal.

What Is "Normal"?

Most of us don't know what "normal" is anymore. Our bodies don't, either, so we get a buildup of cortisol, the long-term stress hormone. Cortisol is essential for heart health, controlling inflammation, and balancing blood-sugar levels, but it can be dangerous when you have elevated levels of it for long periods of time. Over time, excess cortisol leads to adrenal exhaustion, which is charac- terized by fatigue, food cravings, anxiety and insomnia, intolerance to heat and cold, irregular periods, menopausal arthritis, and numerous other symptoms.

Do these sound familiar? They're remarkably similar to the symptoms of perimenopause and menopause. That's no coincidence, since adrenal fatigue and menopause often go hand-in-hand. In the long run, adrenal fatigue caused by unresolved stress can lead to blood-sugar problems, fat accumulation, compromised immune function, exhaustion, bone loss, memory loss, and even heart disease.

Managing Stress

There's no doubt about it. We all need to manage our stress better. It may feel even more stressful to think about ways to manage our stress. We all recognize the pounding heart and racing mind that accompany intense stressors, but what about the smaller stressors that pile up day by day? If we can recognize stress and deal with it as each little stressor comes along, we can avoid the cortisol buildup that leads to big trouble. Here's an easy guide to help you recognize the symptoms of stress:

- Agitation
- Butterflies in stomach
- Irregular breathing
- Irritability
- Muscle tension
- Sudden flush

These sound very much like perimenopausal symptoms, don't they? Since stress, adrenal exhaustion, and menopausal symptoms are so closely related, it stands to reason that they aggravate one another. It also makes sense that managing one of them will help you keep the others in check. Recognizing stress when it occurs gives you the opportunity to deal with it and release it.

Standard medical treatment. Although at least 75 percent of visits to doctors' offices are due to stress-related illness, conventional medicine has little to offer except medications such as high blood-pressure medications, drugs to treat high blood sugar, or pills for migraines. Some doctors may offer anti-anxiety medications or antidepressants, since anxiety and depression often go hand-in-hand with chronic stress, but the medications are frequently ineffective unless the cause of the stress is addressed. And taking these medications can risk serious side effects.

Check your lifestyle. Are you getting enough sleep? Insufficient sleep can lead to elevated blood pressure, weight gain, and irritability—all raising your stress level. Is your diet contributing to good health? Processed and refined foods, sugar, and caffeine all contribute to the stress response. Do you get enough exercise? I know, we have been here before; but exercise literally burns off stress hormones.

Do you take time for yourself? I can guess the answer. Most of us put ourselves last, and our health suffers for the decision. Are you able to say, "No"? When someone asks you for a favor or to take on additional responsibilities, do you know your limits? Do you have a group of friends and family with whom you regularly spend leisure time? Do you laugh together? Cry together? Emotional support and an opportunity for emotional release in a nurturing environment go a long way toward relieving stress.

Some Supplements May Help

There are several effective supplements to help you address toxic stress. The following are among them.

Rhodiola

This Arctic herb actually changes the way your body reacts to stress, making you feel relaxed yet upbeat and alert. Russian animal studies showed that subjects exposed to extreme stress chilled out and improved their performance by 159 percent when they had rhodiola in their systems.

Dosage. Take 100–300 mg daily. The best standardized product is Rosavin, available at some health food stores.

Side effects. Irritability and insomnia have been reported at high doses.

5-HTP

Your body uses 5-hydroxytryptophan (5-HTP) to manufacture the brain chemical serotonin—and a serotonin boost has been shown to alleviate anxiety. It also has a unique way of helping increase your body's natural production of the sleep hormone, melatonin. Studies from the National Institutes of Health (NIH) found that 5-HTP lengthened the amount of time that subjects spent in relaxing rapid-eye movement (REM) sleep by about 25 percent, addressing the insomnia common in perimenopause and helping subjects awaken feeling rested and refreshed.

Dosage. Take 50–100 mg one hour before bedtime. If that's not enough, increase by 50 mg a day until you reach a maximum of 300 mg. The effect is boosted by a vitamin B-complex supplement.

Side effects. Some people experience mild gastrointestinal symptoms after taking 5-HTP.

B Vitamins

Your natural supply of B vitamins is depleted by stress, so supplementation is helpful to improve your ability to make calming hormones and neurotransmitters such as serotonin.

Dosage. Take a B-complex supplement daily. Each dose should supply 100 micrograms (mcg) of vitamin B_{12} and biotin, 400 mcg of folic acid, and 100 mg each of the other B vitamins.

Side effects. None known at the recommended dosage.

GABA

Gamma-aminobutyric acid (GABA) controls the release of the brain-stimulating chemical, dopamine, and cools down racing emotions. Not having enough GABA leads to anxiety, tension, and insomnia, but if you're getting enough, you'll feel tranquil.

Dosage. Take 100–500 mg one to three times daily with meals.

Side effects. Can cause nausea and vomiting at high doses.

Manage Your Time

The biggest stressor for most women is time pressure. You know well that there aren't twenty-five hours in a day. If you feel your life is somehow out of control, try these:

- Keep a to-do list.

- Ask your family for help.

- Schedule a daily appointment with yourself. Allot one hour and then do whatever you want, without interruption. It may require some training for family and friends to leave you alone for this time.

- Schedule weekly social time with friends and family. This is time that doesn't require anyone to clean the house and prepare food. Go out for a coffee date, or walk around the block. Meet at a local park. Sit on someone's front porch. It should be a break for everyone.

- Learn to say, "No."

Years ago, a much revered teacher gave me a benchmark for what's important in the greater scheme of things. It's become a benchmark to measure the drama level of day-to-day stressors. My teacher said, "Ask yourself, 'Will I remember this incident ten years from today?'" If the answer is "yes," then it's important and worth your attention. If the answer is "no," let it go.

What You Can Do

Take time to take a few deep breaths when you feel symptoms of stress. A yoga or tai chi class will give you a number of tools for relieving stress, including slow, sustained stretching and breath control. Finally, meditation, contemplation, prayer—whatever you want to call them, they work. Studies have shown that people who learn to meditate reduce their blood pressure and actually reduce the risk of death from any cause by as much as 23 percent. One study of postmenopausal women who were long-time meditators showed they had one-third the level of cortisol in their urine that nonmeditators did and they had a much lower risk of heart disease.

Meditation

Find a comfortable seated posture with your spine straight. It is fine to sit in a chair, but if you do, be sure to have your feet flat on the floor. If you're sitting on the floor, tuck a cushion under your pelvis to help keep your spine relaxed, but straight. Consciously relax your body. Pay special attention to relaxing the muscles of belly, shoulders, and jaw.

Begin to take deep, slow, regular breaths through your nose, relaxing your belly muscles as you inhale, and slightly contracting them as you exhale. Keep your awareness on the simple inhalation and exhalation. Let your breath find its own rhythm. If your mind wanders, gently bring it back to the breath. Do this for at least ten minutes a day, longer if you like.

Yoga and Tai Chi

The gentle stretching and contemplative movement of some forms of yoga practice and the balanced graceful movement of tai chi, chi gong, and other Eastern disciplines are excellent stress relievers. They're also good ways of toning muscle groups, lowering blood pressure, and improving balance. There are some excellent DVDs available, but as a yoga teacher for many years, I recommend taking at least one course to learn the form of these delightful exercises you like best. A qualified teacher can help you with alignment and pace.

These types of exercise should be approached slowly and gently. Never force yourself into a position. Allow the weight of your body to gently carry you as far as you can go. It may take time to loosen tight muscles, so be gentle with your body. Avoid any teacher or method who insists on forcing you into a position. At the end of a class, you should feel energized, yet relaxed.

CHAPTER 11

BIOIDENTICAL HORMONE REPLACEMENT

Now, you know you are at least perimeno-pausal. You've had the tests done, so you know exactly what's happening in your body—right now. You've got a good diet, and you exercise regularly. You may have tried some of the herbs and supplements I've discussed in this book, but you still aren't satisfied with your results. It's time for the big decision: Do you need hormone replacement therapy (HRT)? If the tests suggest that you do need it, you also need to ask yourself: Do I really want to do that?

The Natural Way

You can rest easy. There are safe and natural ways to duplicate your declining hormones exactly as your body manufactured them in its prime. Your doctor probably won't mention this to you because he or she may not know about these natural hormones that have been available for about thirty years in the United States and since the 1940s in Europe.

Because they are substances natural to the human body, natural hormones can't be patented, so there's little incentive for the pharmaceutical industry to spend the hundreds of millions of dollars required to research and develop them in order to get Food and Drug Administration (FDA) approval. Although early forms were somewhat difficult to use, new technology has made them bioavailable in pills, creams, gels, patches, drops, suppositories, and sublingual tablets.

Bioidentical Hormones

Bioidentical plant-derived progesterone, estradiol, estrone, and testosterone are available through compounding pharmacies that actually formulate the mixture that's best for you based on your test results. You can get natural hormones only by prescription, and their manufacture is standardized. They are regulated by the FDA, contrary to the beliefs of many doctors. Natural hormones are made from highly purified chemicals originally derived from soy and wild yams. A complex manufacturing process transforms them into a carbon copy of the hormones you had at your peak of hormone production.

Many people believe these hormones are natural because they come from plants, but they are actually highly purified pharmaceutical chemicals originally derived from soybeans and wild yams. It's important to note that they are *not* plant or herbal extracts. Through a complex laboratory process, they are converted into actual hormones, making their molecular structures identical to those of the hormones your body makes itself. They are called "natural" because they are identical to your own hormones, not because of their distant plant origins.

Many major pharmaceutical companies are now producing bioidentical hormones, among them the estradiols Estrace, Climara, Vivelle, and Estraderm, and progesterones Prometrium and Crinone. You've made some headway if your doctor wants to prescribe one of these for you, but while they're bioidentical to a hypothetical thirty-five-year old woman, they aren't necessarily customized to you.

Your body has a lock-and-key hormonal structure. To put it simply, your body either manufactures hormones or you take them as supplements, and they fit perfectly into receptors, like keys. Bioidentical hormones fit exactly into those receptors, protecting you against the many dangers of unbalanced hormones. Synthetic hormones don't fit the lock-and-key structure precisely, and some can stay too long or not long enough, worsening your symptoms and increasing your long-term risks.

Natural Hormone Replacement

Dr. Jonathan Wright, one of the pioneers of natural hormone replacement, mentions the following benefits in his book, *Natural Hormone Replacement*:

- Better maintenance of muscle mass and strength
- Far fewer unwanted side effects than synthetic hormones
- Improved cholesterol levels
- Improved libido (sex drive)
- Improved sleep and better mood, concentration, and memory
- Prevention of osteoporosis and restoration of bone strength
- Prevention of senility and Alzheimer's disease
- Protection against heart disease and stroke
- Reduced hot flashes and reduced vaginal dryness and thinning
- Reduced risk of depression
- Reduced risk of endometrial cancer and breast cancer

Bioidentical Estrogen

You can get bioidentical estrogen derivatives in any combination of the following, based on your individual needs:

- Bi-estrogen (estradiol and estriol)
- Tri-estrogen (estrone, estradiol, and estriol)
- Estriol
- Estradiol

Let's look at the pros and cons of each.

Tri-estrogen. This formulation contains one part estradiol to one part estrone to eight parts estriol. Adding small amounts of estradiol and estrone, the most potent estrogen forms, helps to relieve perimenopausal symptoms such as hot flashes and night sweats quickly.

Tri-est helps maintain your hormones at optimal levels. Falling estrogen levels can stimulate estrogen receptors to help replenish reduced levels and, vice versa, it can help lower too-high estrogen levels. One of Tri-est's great beauties is the inclusion of estriol, a well-researched cancer preventive. Tri-est's only drawback is that it may not be strong enough for women in surgical menopause.

Bi-estrogen. Bi-est is usually compounded in a mixture that is 80 percent estriol and 20 percent estradiol. Estrone is left out under the theory that this will minimize the breast cancer risk associated with it.

Estradiol. Although most experts prefer a tri-estrogen formula, plant-derived estradiol combined with progesterone is more effective than a synthetic combination such as Premarin and has the added benefit of reducing fibrocystic changes in the breasts. Estrace, Estraderm, Climara, and Vivelle are natural products based on estradiol alone. A compounding pharmacy can also custom formulate estradiol with a prescription.

Dr. Wright notes that, in the female body, estradiol is always accompanied by estrone and estriol. Furthermore, estradiol is suspected of being the most cancer-causing of any estrogen.

Estriol. Some hormone researchers such as Dr. Wright believe the primary cancer danger from synthetic hormone replacement therapy (HRT) comes not from generalized unopposed estrogen, but from unopposed estradiol, estrone, and equilin.

These are the estrogens found in the urine of pregnant mares, which is used in Premarin. Wright and others believe estriol's role may be to stop the growth of hormone-related cancers.

For years, European doctors have prescribed estriol as a safe and effective alternative to 100 percent estradiol or to premarin. It has been found to be especially helpful for women with disabling menopausal symptoms including vaginal thinning, painful sexual intercourse, recurrent urinary-tract infections, and urinary incontinence. The estriol found in natural hormone replacement is identical to what the body produces naturally.

Estriol has the benefits of stronger estrogens without the risks. Therefore, many European doctors make it the natural hormone replacement of choice. Dr. Marcus Laux says U.S. doctors are "crying out" for estriol's acceptance in this country, but since it cannot be patented, pharmaceutical companies are not interested in it. Compounding pharmacies report an increasing demand for estriol, especially for women who have suffered from breast cancer or are at high risk for it.

The Importance of Progesterone

Although bioidentical hormone replacement is available in the form of estrogen derivatives alone, experts in the field say progesterone replacement is just as important as estrogen replacement—if not more so. Some doctors will tell you that progesterone is necessary only if you have a uterus, so it's not helpful for women who have had a hysterectomy. This is not true!

Progesterone is important to balance unopposed estrogen. It is part of that delicate dance with estrogen. The two are designed to work together, says Dr. Laux. Natural progesterone is part of virtually every natural hormone replacement program. It's important to get natural micronized progesterone, a product that has been processed and refined into tiny, easily absorbed crystals. It is available only by prescription and is vastly different from the wild yam creams available at your health food store.

Testosterone Replacement

If salivary hormone tests show low testosterone levels, you and your doctor might want to consider testosterone replacement. You should be started off with a very low dose, since a tiny amount can have a big impact. Dr. Shari Lieberman says that she has found testosterone to be of greater benefit than either estrogen or progesterone in most cases.

What's Best for You?

It's up to you, your hormone tests, and your doctor to determine what's best for you. The beauty of natural hormone replacement is that you can have a unique formula made just for you, and it can be changed as necessary. It's a good idea to have your hormones retested annually, at least until full menopause. While long-term studies have not been done on natural hormone replacement therapy because it is identical to a woman's natural hormone structure, Dr. Lieberman says that most doctors knowledgeable on the subject are comfortable with advising their menopausal patients to take it for many years.

Finding a Compounding Pharmacy

You need a pharmacist who specializes in compounding (making prescriptions by hand) and titrating (individualizing the dosage). Don't bother to look for this person at your local chain drugstore. To find a compounding pharmacy, call the International Academy of Compounding Pharmacists at (800) 927-4227, ext. 30. It would be best if you could find a compounding pharmacy that specializes in women's health and hormone therapy, but you may have to do some additional footwork to find one. Many excellent compounding pharmacies will work directly with your doctor and send prescriptions through the mail, so it isn't essential that the pharmacy be located close to you.

CONCLUSION

Once you've discovered where you are in the process of perimenopause/menopause, you can choose the way you wish to approach your symptoms and protect your health in the long term. You may have some educating to do, especially with doctors who are unfamiliar with natural approaches to the changes associated with peri-menopause and insurance companies who just "aren't sure."

I hope this book has given you the information you need and the resources to help you make the choices that will work for you with the help of a qualified medical practitioner. Remember: Peri-menopause and menopause are not diseases. They are part of the natural flow of life for every woman. With the healthy and natural approaches offered here, you can live a long and fulfilling life!

SELECTED REFERENCES

Alzheimer's Disease

Keslak, J.P. "Can estrogen play a significant role in the prevention of Alzheimer's disease?" *Journal of Neural Transmission*, 2002; 62 (Supplement): 227–239.

Bone Health

De Souza, M.J., K.M. Prestwood, et al. "A Comparison of the Effect of Synthetic and Micronized Hormone Replacement Therapy on Bone Mineral Density and Biochemical Markers of Bone Metabolism." *Meno-pause: The Journal of the North American Menopause Society*, 1996; 3(3): 140–148.

Lee, J.R. "Osteoporosis reversal: the role of progesterone." *International Clinical Nutrition Review*, 1990; 10(3): 384–391.

Cancer Risk

Ziel, H.K., and W.D. Finkle. "Increased risk of endo-metrial carcinoma among users of conjugated estrogens." *The New England Journal of Medicine*, 1975; 293(23): 1167–1170.

Hormone Replacement

Bassol, S., S. Carranza-Lira, et al. "The impact of a monophasic continuous estro-progestogenic treatment on Latin American menopausal women." *Maturitas*, 2005; 50(3):189–195.

Bilgrami, I., and K. Blower. "Changes in the use of hormone replacement therapy in New Zealand following the publication of the Women's Health Initiative trial." *New Zealand Medical Journal*. 2004 Nov 26;117(1206): U1175.

Cobliegh, M.A., R.F. Berris, et al. for the Breast Cancer Committees of the Eastern Cooperative Oncology

Group. "Estrogen replacement therapy in breast cancer survivors." *Journal of the American Medical Association*, 1994; 272(7): 540–545.

Colditz, G.A., S.E. Hankinson, et al. "The use of estrogens and progestins and the risk of breast cancer in post-menopausal women." *The New England Journal of Medicine*, 1995; 332: 1589–1593.

Folsom, A. et al. "Hormonal replacement therapy and morbidity and mortality in a prospective study of post-menopausal women." *American Journal of Public Health*, 1995; 85(8): 1128(5).

Hargrove, J.T., W. Maxson, et al. "Menopausal hormone replacement therapy with continuous daily oral micronized estradiol and progesterone." *Obstetrics and Gynecology*, 1989; 73: 606–612.

Hargrove, J.T., K.G. Oseen, et al. "An alternative method of hormone replacement therapy using natural sex steroids." *Menopause: The Journal of the North American Menopause Society*, 1995; 6:653–674.

Lemon, H.M. "Estriol, the forgotten estrogen?" *Journal of the American Medical Association*, 1978; 239(1): 29–30.

Ottoson, E., et al. "Al. Subfractions of high density lipoprotein cholesterol during estrogen replacement therapy: a comparison between progestins and natural progesterone." *Journal of Obstetrics and Gynecology* 151 (1985): 746–750.

Hormone Testing

Ellison, P. "Measurement of Salivary Progesterone." *Annals of the New York Academy of Sciences*, 1992: 161–176.

Nutrition

Lushi, L.K., et al. "Dietary antioxidant vitamins and death from coronary artery disease in postmenopausal women." *New England Journal of Medicine*, 1996; 334(18): 11556–11562.

Plant Estrogens

Beckman, N. "Phyto-oestrogens and compounds that effect oestrogen metabolism, parts I and II." *Australian Journal of Medical Herbalism*, 1995; 7:11–23.

Progesterone

Chakmakjian, A.H., and N.Y. Zachariah. "Bioavailability of progesterone with different modes of administration." *The Journal of Reproductive Medicine*, 1987; 32(6): 443–447.

De Lignieres, B. "Effects of progestrogens on the postmenopausal breast." *Climacteric*, 2002; 5(3): 229–235.

Stress

Schneider, R.H., C.N. Alexander, et al. "Long-term effects of stress reduction on mortality in persons >/=55 years of age with systemic hypertension." *American Journal of Cardiology*, 2005 May 1; 95(9): 1060–1064.

Trigo, M., D. Silva, et al. "Psychosocial risk factors in coronary heart disease: beyond type A behavior." *Review Portuguese Cardiology*, 2005 Feb; 24(2): 261–281.

Women's Health Initiative

American College of Obstetricians and Gynecologists. *Questions and Answers on Hormone Therapy: In Response to the Women's Health Initiative Study Results on Estrogen and Progestin.* (Washington, D.C., American College of Obstetricians and Gynecologists, August 2002).

OTHER BOOKS AND RESOURCES

Books

Ahlgrimm, Marla, and John M. Kells. *The HRT Solution* (Avery, 1999).

Estes, Clarissa Pinkola. *Women Who Run with the Wolves* (Ballantine, 1996).

Laux, Marcus, and Christine Conrad. *Natural Woman, Natural Menopause* (Harper Collins, 1997).

Lee, John, Jesse Hanley, and Virginia Hopkins. *What Your Doctor May Not Tell You About Premenopause: Balance Your Life and Your Hormones from Thirty to Fifty* (Warner Books 1999).

Lieberman, Shari. *Get Off the Menopause Roller Coaster* (Avery, 2000).

Northrup, Christiane. *The Wisdom of Menopause* (Bantam, 2001).

Reiss, Uzzi. *Natural Hormone Therapy for Women* (Atria, 2002).

Wright, Jonathan, and John Morgenthaler. *Natural Hormone Replacement for Women Over 45* (Smart Publications, 1997).

Magazines

GreatLife Magazine
Consumer magazine with articles on vitamins, minerals, herbs, and foods.
Available for free at many health and natural food stores.

Let's Live Magazine
Consumer magazine with emphasis on the health benefits of vitamins, minerals, and herbs.
Customer service:
1-800-676-4333
P.O. Box 74908
Los Angeles, CA 90004

Subscriptions: 12 issues per year, $19.95 in the U.S.;
$31.95 outside the U.S.

Physical Magazine

Magazine oriented to body builders and other serious athletes.
Customer service:
1-800-676-4333
P.O. Box 74908
Los Angeles, CA 90004
Subscriptions: 12 issues per year, $19.95 in the U.S.;
$31.95 outside the U.S.

The Nutrition Reporter™ newsletter

Monthly newsletter that summarizes recent medical research on vitamins, minerals, and herbs.
Customer service:
P.O. Box 30246
Tucson, AZ 85751-0246
e-mail: jack@thenutritionreporter.com
www.nutritionreporter.com
Subscriptions: $26 per year (12 issues) in the U.S.; $32 U.S.
or $48 CNC for Canada; $38 for other countries

Referrals

Women's International Pharmacy: www.womensinter national.com will send you an information packet and a list of doctors in your area who have prescribed through their service.

Women's Health America and Madison Pharmacy Associates (founded by Marla Ahlgrimm): www.womens health.com has an excellent reference section and can supply bioidentical hormones, as well as free follow-up testing to be sure your dosage is accurate.

Saliva Hormone Testing and Urine Bone-Loss Testing

Aeron Life Cycles Clinical Laboratory
www.aeron.com
Phone: 1-800-631-7900

Websites

Crone Chronicles: www.cronechronicles.com

Susun Weed: www.menopause-metamorphosis.com with practical suggestions for addressing changes in body, mind, and spirit.

INDEX

Acetylcholine, 35
Adrenal glands, 28, 30
Adrenal exhaustion, 28,
    69–70
Aging, 24–26
Ahlgrimm, Marla, 9, 14, 29,
    32
Alcohol, 43
Alpha lipoic acid (ALA), 61
Altrazine, 12
Alzheimer's disease, 2, 15,
    30, 34–35
Anemia, 44
Antioxidants, 33
Ascorbic acid. See Vitamin C.

Beta-carotene, 51
Bi-estrogen, 79
Bioidentical hormone
    replacement, 76–82
Biotin, 51
Black cohosh (Cimecifuga
    racemosa), 23, 52
Blood pressure, 28, 31
Blood tests, 16–20
Bone, 33–34
    density, 44
    supplements for, 56–58
Boron, 34, 51, 57–58
Brain function, supplements
    for, 59–61
Breast swelling, 10
Broccoli, 36

Caffeine, 43
Calcium, 34, 36, 51, 56
Cancer, 2, 30, 31–33
    breast, 5, 32, 39, 44
    cervical, 32
    colon, 15
    endometrial, 5
    hormone-related, 32
    ovarian, 5, 32
    uterine, 23, 32
Chemicals, 12, 33
Chi gong, 48
Cholesterol, high-density
    (HDL), 31

Chromium, 51, 62
Climara, 77, 79
Cobalamin. See Vitamin B$_{12}$.
Coenyzme Q$_{10}$, 54
Coffee. See Caffeine.
Compounding pharmacies,
    81–82
Conventional medicine,
    21–23, 70–71
Copper, 51
Cortisol, 16, 18, 69
Crinone, 77
Crone Chronicles, 8

Dairy products, 42
Damiana (Turnera diffusa,
    aphrodisiaca), 64–64
DDT, 12
Depression, supplements
    for, 59–61
Dehydroepiandrosterone.
    See DHEA.
Dental changes, 5
Depression, 4–5, 7, 19, 23,
    71
DHEA, 16, 26, 31, 34, 55
    test levels, 17–18
Diabetes, type 2, 2
Dichloro-diphenyl-trichloro -
    methane. See DDT.
Diet, 24–25, 33, 36–43. See
    also Food.
Diethylstilbestrol (DES), 12
Doctors, 13–20
Dong quai (Angelica
    sinensis), 55
Dopamine, 35
Drugs, 12

EFAs, 40
Emotional health, 67–71
Endometrial cells, 9–10
Endosulphan, 12
Equilin, 22, 79
Essential fatty acids. See
    EFAs.
Estrace, 77, 79
Estraderm, 77, 79

Estradiol, 15, 22, 26, 39, 77
  bioidentical, 79
  test levels, 17
Estriol, 15, 22, 39, 79–80
Estrogen, 1–2, 4, 6, 9–11,
    14–15, 18, 26, 27, 30–35,
    38, 45, 78–80
  equine, 6, 21–23, 35
  excess, 28
  toxic, 11–12
  unopposed, 32
Estrogen receptors, 34–35
Estrone, 15, 22, 77, 79
Evening primrose oil
    (*Oenothera biennis*),
    55–56
Exercise, 24–25, 34, 44–49
Extremeties, cold, 19
Eyebrows, thinning, 19

Fatigue, 19
Fats, 33, 40
Fatty tissue, 11–12
Fiber, 37
Fibrinogen, 31
Fish, 40
Fight or flight, 68–69
5-HTP, 72
Flour, white, 41
Fluid retention, 10
Folate. *See* Folic acid.
Folic acid, 51
Follicle-stimulating
    hormone, 10
Food, 36–43
  basic rules, 41–43
  colorful, 37, 41
  cravings, 5
  fried, 42
  junk, 41–42
  natural, 41
  See also Diet.
Fosamax, 14, 34
Fruits, 33, 37, 41

GABA, 73
Gardening, 46
Garlic (*Allium sativum*), 58
*Get Off the Menopause
    Roller Coaster,* 6, 36
Ginkgo (*Ginkgo biloba*), 59,
    65
Glutamine, 62
Grains, whole, 33, 41

Hair, 5 19
HCA (*Garcinia cambogia*),
    62–63
Headaches, 4–5, 10
Heart attacks, 2, 30–31
Heart disease, 5, 15, 23,
    30–31, 44
  supplements to prevent,
    58–59
  symptoms, 30–31
Heart rate, 47
Heavy metals. *See* Metals,
    heavy.
Herbicides, 12
Herbs, 25, 50–66
High-density lipoprotein
    (HDL). *See* Cholesterol.
Homocysteine, 31
Hormone replacement
    therapy (HRT), 1–3, 6–7,
    10, 21–23, 35, 36, 38,
    76–82
Hormones, 1–3, 4–8, 9–12, 44
  natural, 76–82
  testing for levels, 14, 16–20
Hot flashes, 1, 4–5, 23, 30
HRT Solution, The, 9, 29, 32
Human growth hormone, 45
Hydroxycitric acid. *See* HCA.
Hypothyroidism, 18–19

Immune system, 44
Indole-3 carbinol, 37
Inositol, 51
Insecticides, 12
Insomnia, 1, 5
Isothiocyanates, 37
Insurance, 20
Iodine, 51
Irritability, 4–5, 7, 19, 30

Joint pain, 4–5
*Journal of the American
    Medical Association,* 50
Junk food, 41–42

Kava kava (*Piper
    methysticum*), 59–60
Kreilkamp, Ann, 8

Lab tests, 16–20
L-carnitine, 54–55, 62
Laux, Marcus, 14, 33, 34, 38,
    80

Lee, John, 14
Libido, 26, 29
Lieberman, Shari, 6, 14, 36, 50, 81
Lifestyle, 71
Liver, 28
Luteinizing hormone, 10

Maca (*Lepidium meyenii*), 64
Magnesium, 34, 51, 56–57
Manganese, 34, 51
Meat, 42
Meditation, 75
Memory loss, 1, 5, 19, 44
Menopause, 1–3, 5–8, 9–12, 13–20, 21–23, 24–26, 27–35, 38, 40–41, 50–66, 67–75, 76–82, 83
  artificial, 11
  average age of, 5, 7, 27
  natural, 11
  natural approaches to, 13–14
  premature, 11
  risks, 30
  spiritual element of, 7–8
  supplements for, 52
  symptoms, 24–26
  timeline, 29
  types of, 11
Menstrual cycles, 5, 19
Menstruation, 4, 10
Metals, heavy, 12
Minerals, 51
Mood swings, 1, 5, 7, 23, 30

Natural Hormone Replace - ment for Women Over 45, 14, 78
Natural killer cells (NK), 32
Natural Woman, Natural Menopause, 33
Niacin. *See* Vitamin B₃.
Night sweats, 1, 5
Noradrenaline, 35
Northrup, Christiane, 11, 14, 18, 26, 29, 67

Oils, 40
  seed, 42
Olive oil, 40–42
Osteopenia, 33
Osteoporosis, 5, 15, 23, 25, 30, 33–34

Ovaries, 27

Palpitations, 5
Pantothenic acid, 51
Para-aminobenzoic acid (PABA), 51
Perimenopause, 4–8, 9–11, 15, 18, 20, 21–23, 24, 27, 29, 38–39, 50–66, 67–75, 76–82
  length of time of, 6
  supplements for, 52–56
  symptoms, 5
  timeline, 29
Periodontal changes, 5
Periods, menstrual, 5, 10
Pesticides, 12
Pharmacies, compounding, 81–82
Phosphorus, 34
Phytoestrogens, 39
Phytohormones, 39
Phytonadione. *See* Vitamin K.
Pinkola Estés, Clarissa, 7
Plastics, 12
Policosanol, 58–59
Pollution, 12
Postmenopause, 27–35
Premarin, 14, 21–22, 35, 79–80
PremPro, 21
Progesterone, 4, 9–10, 15, 22–23, 26, 31–33, 38, 77, 80–81
  bioidentical, 77, 80–81
  synthetic, 35
  syptoms of declining, 10
  test levels, 17
Progestin, 22
Prometrium, 77
Provera, 14
Pyridoxine. *See* Vitamin B₆.

Red clover (*Trifolium pratense*), 53–54
Relaxation, 68–69
Rhodiola, 71
Riboflavin. *See* Vitamin B₂.

S-adenosyl methionine (SAM-e), 60
Saliva testing, 20
Salt, 43

SAM-e. *See* S-adenosyl
    methionine (SAM-e).
Seed oils, 42
Selenium, 51
Serotonin, 35
Sex, 5, 25–26
Sex drive, supplements for,
    64–65
Skin, 44
    dry, 19
    elasticity, 5
Sleep, 72
Smoking, 33
Sodas, 43
Soy, 38, 39
Soy isoflavones, 52
St. John's wort, 61
Strength training, 48
Stress, 33, 67–75
    lifestyle and, 71
    managing, 70–71, 73–75
    standard medical
        treatment, 70–71
Strokes, 2, 23
Sugar, 43
Sulforaphane, 37
Supplements, 25, 50–66,
    71–73
    for depression and brain
        function, 59–61
    for heart disease, 58
    for perimenopause and
        menopause, 52–56
    for sex drive, 64–65
    for strong bones, 56–58
    for weight control, 61–64
    how to use, 65–66

Tai chi, 48, 74–75
Testosterone, 15, 26, 31, 34,
    44–45, 77, 81
    dropping levels, 29
    replacement, 29
    test levels, 17
Thiamine. *See* Vitamin B_1.
Thymus gland, 10
Thyroid, 18–20, 28
    lab tests for function,
        18–19
    low function symptoms, 19
Thyroid-stimulating
    hormone, 18–19
    test, 18–19
Thyroxine, 19

Time management, 73
Timelines, 29
Tooth decay, 15
Toxins, 33, 39
Tri-estrogen, 79
Trimethylglycine (TMG), 60

Urinary incontinence, 5, 15

Vaginal dryness and itching, 5
Vanderhaeghe, Lorna, 27
Vegetables, 33, 36–39, 41
    cruciferous, 39
Vitamin A, 36, 51
Vitamin B complex, 51, 72
Vitamin B_1, 51
Vitamin B_2, 51
Vitamin B_3, 51
Vitamin B_6, 51
Vitamin B_{12}, 51
Vitamin C, 36, 51
Vitamin D, 34, 51
Vitamin D_3, 57
Vitamin E, 51
Vitamin K, 34, 57
Vitamins, multi, with
    minerals, 36, 50–51
Vitex (*Vitex agnus castus*),
    23, 53
Vivelle, 77, 79

Walking, 45–47
Water retention, 10, 23
Weight
    gain, 5, 10, 19, 39–40
    loss, 19
Weight-bearing exercise, 45
Weight control,
    supplements for, 61–64
Whey protein, 63–64
*Wisdom of Menopause,
    The*, 11
*Women Who Run with the
    Wolves*, 7
Women's Health Initiative, 2,
    7, 21, 35
Wright, Jonathan, 14, 22, 78,
    79

Xenoestrogens, 11–12, 27

Yoga, 48, 74–75

Zinc, 51

9 781681 628639